CALL THE
PHARMACIST

Elizabeth Roddick F.R.Pharm.S

To Ann

Best wishes

Elizabeth Roddick

CALL THE PHARMACIST

First published in 2013 by

Panoma Press

48 St Vincent Drive, St Albans, Herts, AL1 5SJ, UK

info@panomapress.com

www.panomapress.com

Book layout by Charlotte Mouncey

Printed on acid-free paper from managed forests.

ISBN 978-1-909623-24-8

This book is dedicated to my late parents,
my patients and customers

Acknowledgements

With thanks to my husband Douglas, Joy Adamson, Laura Borland, Brenda Bree, Liz Grant, Dr Gordon Jefferson, Dr John McKay, Dr Howard McNulty, Anne Murray, Kay Roberts, Jennifer Strong, Angela Timoney and Janie Vickers.

Contents

Introduction

'You've got two days to clear your things out of the shop'. That was the stark phone call my father received when he was manager of the tiny chemist shop opposite the Toledo picture house in Clarkston Road, south Glasgow. It was 1938 and he had always been told in the past that he would get a fair chance to buy the business from the non-pharmacy owners when they decided to sell, but that was clearly not to be. Nowadays, there would be industrial tribunals, hearings and compensation.

My parents had just got married and had taken out a large loan from the bank to buy their house (there were no mortgages in those days) so to receive a telephone call like that must have been devastating. My father initially tried working for another pharmacist – a Mr Hunter in the next row of shops down – but that didn't work out. I suspect my mother then took charge of the situation and encouraged him to go out on his own. So, about a month later, he decided to take the plunge and open up his own pharmacy, 'James M. Ure Chemist', in Cathcart. What was just so rewarding was that many of his patients followed him down the road to help him in what was a precarious situation.

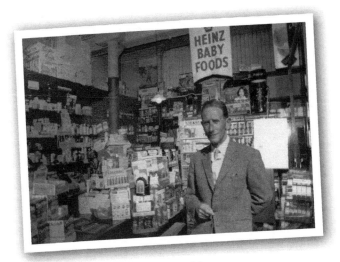

Mr Jimmy Ure

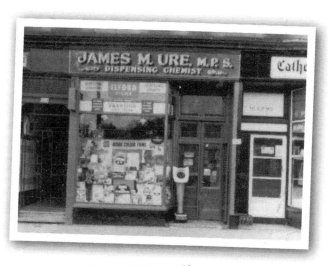

James M. Ure Chemist

My father, as a 'chemist', was needed at home during the war. In his professional capacity, he always had a plentiful supply of restricted commodities such as large bottles of syrup and tea. Many a 'barter' took place with each person bringing his or her own speciality to the transaction.

As the war ended, the baby boom began and, because there were no large supermarkets at that time, the chemist's shop became the place to get everything. My father's shop was the centre for 'new mum' advice where every baby was weighed (sometimes on a weekly basis) and as the babies grew, he had the knack of encouraging the children in with a plentiful supply of lollipops.

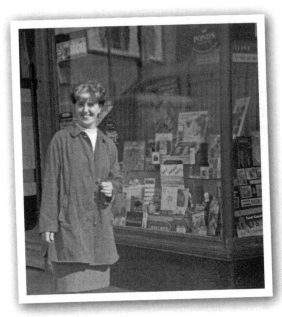

His trusty assistant, Betty Shields, was off the same block and would make such a fuss of the babies and toddlers that the young mums would laugh and beam with pride whenever they visited. She was known as 'Betty in the Chemist' and even today, in her eighties, some of 'her babies' still recognise her and call her by that name.

On her retirement, she was presented with two tickets for a trip on Concorde.

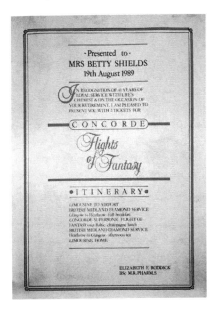

My father was always immaculately dressed with a three-piece suit, collar and tie but behind that professional exterior there lurked a dry, mischievous sense of humour.

I can remember three occasions to illustrate this. The first was when a lady called in and asked for a particular colour of toilet roll that my father did not stock. My father retorted with a wry smile, 'You'll be wanting a tartan one next!' The lady turned and left. She didn't appreciate my father's sense of fun.

The second example was when a representative from a particular company was checking stock and said to my father in a rather worried voice, 'I'm afraid Mr Ure, it looks as if you have had some stock stolen.'

'Oh well,' said my father 'it always keeps the stock down.' The representative laughed heartily and used to use that story at many a meeting afterwards.

The third time my father's sense of humour was evident almost got him into trouble with the local medical profession. A gentleman had called in and handed over a prescription. Without looking up he retorted 'It looks like a hen has walked over the prescription, what a mess!' He then looked up and saw to his horror this was actually the particular GP standing in front of him. The GP looked him straight in the eye and said, 'I see I'm going to have to write much more clearly in *this* district.'

But something happened to my father that changed his life dramatically.

It was one Saturday night in 1974 when he was walking back to the house when he was set upon by two thugs. They knocked him to the ground and kicked him in the face and body. They knew he had the shop takings and they hooted with laughter as they ran away with the brown package they had forced from his pocket. It was in fact a packet of soap that my father was taking round to a friend's house that night. The thieves had got nothing from the robbery but they did inflict pain and suffering needlessly.

That episode had a dramatic effect on my father's life. From that day he didn't seem to have the same confidence to enjoy his games of bowls up at Cathcart Bowling Club. Although his sense of humour was still evident, he started to lose his short-term memory.

We will never know whether that episode shortened his life but sadly, he died in 1995 at the age of 87. His memory still lives on in those that knew him and benefited from his wise counsel.

But it was the lure of that special smell, a mixture of perfume and surgical spirit along with the rows of brightly coloured bottles with liquids and powders that fascinated me growing up. When these ingredients were miraculously turned into medicinal compounds, the fascination with chemistry and science grew.

At a later stage, I was allowed to mix powders using a mortar and pestle and then to formulate ointments on a large slab with a spatula. Yes, I was hooked. There was nothing else I wanted to do – I was going to be a pharmacist.

And so I took my degree at Strathclyde University and after a year at the Victoria Infirmary, followed by various managerial positions, I decided that building up relationships with patients and customers was the most satisfying part of my work and I could only do that if I was permanently in one place. In 1982, I decided to buy my father's business and it was renamed E.F.Ure Pharmacy.

I had only just settled into the pharmacy when a chance meeting with a surveyor friend resulted in my finding out that seven pharmacists had heard about the doctor's surgery moving up to the old police building. The pharmacists were all after premises just down the road from my pharmacy and if they had succeeded in acquiring them, my business would have closed. I quickly phoned my lawyer and managed to secure the lease on the old fish shop opposite the proposed surgery site and, with a sigh of relief I got ready to move my business down the road.

One year later, when pharmacies could open anywhere they wished, I heard that another pharmacist was going to open about 50 yards from where I was situated.

I decided to go and see the other pharmacist to explain that two pharmacies could not exist side by side but he went ahead and opened anyway.

That was when I decided to start my delivery service and I also opened right through the lunch hour, Sundays and public holidays. We had set up a spy across the road who would phone us every time the other pharmacy opened outside the normal times and either my father or myself went down and opened up our own premises.

Every week I managed to find a story about my pharmacy or indeed a family story such as my parents' golden wedding anniversary where they went round the world, in order to focus attention on the business

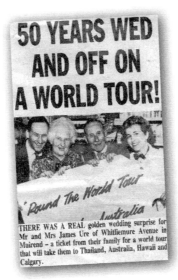

50 YEARS WED AND OFF ON A WORLD TOUR!

"Round The World Tour"

Australia

THERE WAS A REAL golden wedding surprise for Mr and Mrs James Ure of Whitliemure Avenue in Muirend – a ticket from their family for a world tour that will take them to Thailand, Australia, Hawaii and Calgary.

Five months later, with a notice in the other pharmacy's window saying, 'sale to make way for Christmas stock' they closed their doors.

In a sense it really helped me establish the business, but during those five months I had many sleepless nights.

In 1985 I got the chance to buy the premises next door and incorporated two consulting rooms, one for chiropody and the other for my own consultations where my patients needed some extra privacy.

So I ran my business for 26 years getting to know my patients and being involved with their families. At one point I was dealing with three generations of customers and so, when I realised that my health was being affected by trying to run two pharmacies, (by this time I had opened my present pharmacy, New Life Pharmacy in Netherlee), I decided to sell E.F.Ure Pharmacy. I didn't want to sell in an open market because I wanted to make sure that my patients were well looked after, so I approached a colleague and asked him if he would like to buy my business.

I had booked a month's trip away at the beginning of February to New Zealand so I thought it would work well if the 1st February 2008 was the date of the sale.

Because of the confidentiality clause in the sale I was unable to tell anyone until very late in the proceedings. The first task was to tell my staff and that was difficult since some of them had been with me for many years. Reassuring them that their jobs were secure did help, but it was still a shock that change was going to happen and that it was happening very quickly.

As far as my patients were concerned I couldn't speak about it, first of all, in case anyone changed allegiance and came to my new pharmacy – that wouldn't be fair – but also, it was like a bereavement. Building up relationships with people for 26 years is not something that can be forgotten.

I still miss many of my former patients and just hope they understand how I could not say I was leaving but also, that I do still miss them and wish them well.

My life in pharmacy started with the role model of my father. After becoming a pharmacist myself and not long into my career, I decided I was going to dedicate my life to pharmacy. I made a promise to myself. I was not only going to be the best pharmacist I could be, but also I would promote the profession at all levels through my work. It was as if a rocket had been lit inside my body. I was going to propel my own practice and that of the profession to the highest heights possible. This book tells the story of the great variety of patient care in the community setting, the development of pharmacy services over the last thirty years and how my life unfolded within that context.

CHAPTER 1
HOME VISITS

Hepler in 1990 [1] described something called pharmaceutical care plans. He suggested that a patient's quality of life could be improved by 'the responsible provision of drug therapy'. In 1994 I decided to do my own 'plans' with my patients and a record of that was published [2]. It seemed to me that pharmacists could take on the responsibility of sorting out old out-of-date medicines and liaising with GPs and other healthcare professionals about any drug-related problems.

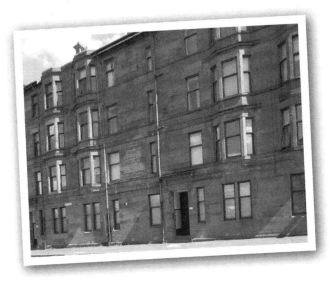

Glasgow Tenements

I don't know what it is about the Glasgow 'close'. The close is the name given to the entrance to a tenement building. Glasgow tenements are four storey sandstone structures that were built during the early 20th century to provide housing to the burgeoning population at that time. You are quite often 'stuck' outside talking to an imaginary person through an intercom. They never had controlled entries in the early days and many a courtship blossomed as a result of this semi-private area away from the prying eyes of nosey neighbours.

The 'control' part of the entrance was the problem. It had to be opened by the person inside and if they happened to be 85 years old and deaf then you could be spending some time on the pavement. It was of course lashing rain and I had had my finger pressing the bell for some time. There was no answer. I knew Sadie was there because I had telephoned to tell her I was popping in to check over her medicines and to find out how she was feeling today. Sadie had heart failure and research had shown that there are fewer hospital visits and better control of symptoms if patients are followed up on a regular basis. Heart failure nurses are the mainstay of this service but because community pharmacists tend to be dealing with these patients on often a monthly basis, it has been found that pharmacists can also play an important part. [3]

Five minutes into my ordeal of trying to get in, a middle-aged woman arrived and opened the outside door. At least I was inside, soaking but sheltered from the elements. I asked if she knew Mrs Conner and she replied, 'You mean Sadie? She's in number 654, that's next door. My you look fair drookit! Would you like a wee cup of tea?'

Thankfully, the rain had elongated my fringe partly covering my face so the kind neighbour in front of me didn't see the embarrassed flush covering my cheeks. How could I be so stupid as to be trying to rouse the wrong person? At least that inhabitant had been out, since sometimes the retort you received when pressing the wrong number was choice!

'No thank you,' I managed to stutter before heading out the door again. I went up to the next close and this time I checked the number on the heart failure documentation. (Thankfully I'd put the paperwork in a 'polypak' sleeve, otherwise it would have been unreadable with the rain soaking my case).

Pressing the bell, I waited. Eighty-five year olds with heart failure take a long time to answer but eventually Sadie shouted 'Hello, who's there?' 'It's Elizabeth Roddick the chemist.' 'Come away in' said Sadie.

This is the tricky part because unless the person inside presses the button, nothing is going to release the outside door. No, it didn't budge. Maybe if I tried a neighbour they could open the outside door and I would be in.

I was still standing outside a few minutes later when I suddenly realised that Sadie was making her way along the corridor towards the outside door. She had come out of her flat and was attempting to make it to the close entrance. When I say 'make it' I was quite concerned because heart failure patients can become very short of breath with exertion and I wondered if I would be calling an ambulance as opposed to conducting a routine visit. No, she was able to let me in and after a wee rest, we headed back to her flat arm-in-arm.

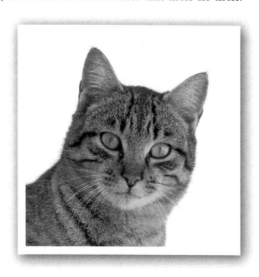

We were met by Sheba the cat and of course introductions and petting had to be performed before we could get down to the business of the assessment. The walk inside the close entrance allowed me to assess Sadie for her breathing and ability to walk. She was quite 'wabbit' (or fatigued) when she sat down and I let her sit for a few minutes before asking her some questions.

'So how are you getting on with your medicines?' I asked. 'Fine, except I don't take my water tablet on a Tuesday because that's the day my friend Elsie takes me out for my shopping.' 'What time does she come for you?' I asked. 'Ten o'clock sharp' said Sadie.

I marvelled at some of these elderly patients who could rattle off all the names of their medicines and what they were for but of course not all patients are in the same league as Sadie. 'You know it would be best to take your water tablet every day. Could you take it when you come back?' 'I suppose I could' said Sadie.

I had noted her ankles were quite puffy looking and I asked if Sadie had noticed that herself. This is one of the physical signs of worsening heart failure so I wanted to make sure that she had been taking her tablets every day and whether her ankles felt a bit swollen to her.

'Yes, I suppose they have got a bit bigger. I find I can't get my stockings on some days and my home help often has a struggle with them. We usually end up laughing.' After I had completed the other question and answers to do with symptoms of heart failure, I told Sadie that I was going to contact her doctor to tell him about her ankles and the suggestion that she should take two of her water tablets for a few days.

'Help, I'll never be off the toilet, dear' retorted Sadie. 'It's just for a few days to see if that makes a difference to your ankles and remember, you can take the tablets at lunchtime next Tuesday.'

I noticed from the care summary that the community nurse was calling in the next day to give Sadie her B12 injection (for her pernicious anaemia) so I made a mental note to leave a message for her about the extra dose when I telephoned the surgery. After saying my necessary farewells to Sheba and checking again that Sadie understood what was going to happen, I headed out into the pouring rain.

I'd only got outside the close when my mobile rang. It was Trish from the pharmacy. She sounded quite frantic. 'It's Mr Foster, he's demanding his medicine and it doesn't matter what we say he's still standing shouting at the top of his voice.'

We used to call Mr Foster 'the colonel' because although he was only five foot four inches tall, he commanded such authority in his voice that when he came in, it was like standing by your dispensing bench, getting ready for inspection. He had been with us for many years but unfortunately, like many articulate people, his short-term memory and subsequently his ability to think rationally had gradually left him as he aged.

'Trish, sit him down in one of the consulting rooms with the phone and, in approximately five minutes time, come in and tell Mr Foster that his daughter has been calling and was worried that he wasn't at home. Can you phone his daughter on the other phone and let her know what has happened? Thanks.' I waited, knowing how much time it would take to lead him into the consulting room and yes, holding the phone away from my ear, I started the conversation. 'Mr Foster, it's good to talk with you today. How are you?' 'Well I'm not well at all. Do you know that I haven't received my medication all week?'

'That's strange, I replied 'because my driver Alan has your signature on our delivery sheet where you personally signed for your medicine two days ago–last Tuesday.' There was silence for a moment as that revelation sunk in. 'You must be mistaken

Mrs Roddick because I was away all day Tuesday at my daughter's'.

'We're just checking with your daughter right now because it is a very serious matter if you say you haven't had your medication when we assure you that you have.' I could feel Mr Foster's tone softening slightly since I could now hold the phone a little closer to my ear and as we argued back and forth, I wish I'd said to Trish to make it two minutes. Suddenly, I could hear a second voice. Trish was excusing herself and letting Mr Foster know that his daughter was making her way to his home and he needed to return quickly.

Panic over, Trish told me on the phone that Mr Foster had apologised he couldn't speak to me anymore since he had been 'summoned' by a higher power. 'Thanks Trish, any other problems let me know.'

I'd managed to get myself into the car to take the call so at least I was sheltered from the elements. I then made the call to Sadie's doctor's surgery. Hilary, the receptionist, took a note of my suggestion and asked if I would like to speak to Dr Douglas since it was the end of his surgery. 'Yes, put me through Hilary.'

I explained what I had discussed with Sadie and he agreed but, like many of my conversations with the local doctors, he had a question for me. 'I've got this patient on a drug for epilepsy but I need to give it in liquid form what do you suggest?' After noting the name and dose of the drug, I explained that I was in my car but would get back to him before his afternoon surgery.

I looked at my next visit. This wasn't going to be so pleasant. It was a lady who felt she was totally in command of her medicine but, because she had ended up in hospital with a suspected over-dose, the GP had asked if her medication could be placed in a weekly tray or compliance aid, as it's called. These compliance aids are the bane of pharmacists' lives.

Instead of dispensing patients' medication in calendar (28 or 30) day packs from the manu-facturer, our dispensers or technicians spend hours popping tablets and capsules out of the original packs. They are then re-dispensed into seven day blister packs marked with the times of taking - breakfast, lunch, tea and bedtime. This means that the patient, usually prompted by a carer, takes the medication at the right time. This process adds literally hours a week to the normal working of the pharmacy and then, to top it all, when a dose is changed mid-week, the tray has to brought back from the patient, revamped or completely renewed and then re-delivered.

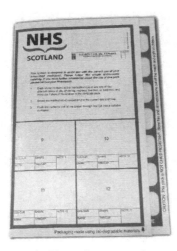

A Compliance Aid

However, what these packs have enabled people to do is to allow them to live in their own homes whereas before, they would probably have needed to be looked after in a residential home with a huge increase in cost to the government. For new patients, training carers to dispense from original containers with medication sheets for initialling when a carer gives a medicine seems the sensible way forward.

I looked at the paperwork for the compliance aid assessment for my next visit. The patient's name was Martha McGregor and she lived in one of the sheltered housing complexes nearby. It was a tiny house but had been kept meticulously. I observed even the climbing roses had a symmetry about them as if the owner had spent many years pruning and willing the plant to grow in a certain direction.

I had been told that her son would be there and I had checked with the warden, Alison, whether it would be a good idea for her to pop in as well and that was when I received the warning. 'This lady is certainly not used to interference in her affairs' said Alison. Wardens, I've found over the years generally have hearts of gold. They care for their residents almost as if they were their own parents and have such a wealth of knowledge, they are invaluable when getting involved with patients in their patch.

'Hello Mrs McGregor' (no first names in this instance) was met with a steely 'Hello, come in, my son is already here. I don't know why, mind you.' I was led into a small lounge that again reflected the immaculate nature of the owner. Mrs McGregor had 'everything in its place.' There was nothing of the clutter that some homes (including my own) have, filling every available space.

'Dr Messer, (always a good idea to start with the reason I was there including the doctor's name, in other words on this occasion, it wasn't my idea.), Dr Messer has asked me to call to discuss how to make your medicines safer.' 'Well I suppose if Dr Messer has said for you to come, I'd better listen to what you have to say.'

We sat round the coffee table. Mrs McGregor taking charge of the meeting with her son on her right and I took the left-hand position so that I could see all the medication that had been gathered in the middle. It's usually at this point that I find old out-of-date medicines or dozens of packets of a 'when required' medicine like paracetamol which the patient thought they were to order every month. It's also a good idea to ask if all the medicines are out of drawers. Many older patients keep medicines secreted away – 'just in case.' This was not so with Mrs McGregor. Everything seemed to be in order.

The compliance aid assessment takes about half an hour and involves asking the patient if, firstly, they know what the medications are for and when they are taking them. Mrs McGregor, although speaking in a staccato, monosyllabic style, answered my questions perfectly. With each answer, I looked across at her son David for reassurance that, yes, his mother did know what was happening. Often a patient will 'put on a face' for the health professional and it's only afterwards that you realise things weren't as they seemed.

It was when we discussed the ordering and procuring of the prescriptions that Mrs McGregor admitted that things hadn't been working too well. 'And I don't want to be bothering David with getting my prescriptions. He's got too much to do,' she retorted. The assessment was over and I wrote my findings in a note to Dr Messer on the back of the form. Mrs McGregor did not need a compliance aid. She did however require a pick up prescription service from the surgery that my driver would be happy to do. We could also deliver back to her home. I also stated we would monitor the time intervals between prescription ordering in case she was asking for her prescriptions too early or late.

I said my goodbyes to Mrs McGregor but I noticed her son 'eyeballing' me. 'Could I have a word with you outside Mrs Roddick?' 'Certainly' I said and stepped out of the house.

I could hear the tension in David McGregor's voice and when we got outside he turned on me. 'I thought my mother was to get a weekly tray?' he stated abruptly. 'Dr Messer thought it might be helpful but, having performed the assessment, that is not the answer for your mother. I suggest we monitor your mother over the next few weeks. Perhaps you can also ask her about her medication each time you call in?'

He started to relent when I added 'Your mother is an intelligent woman. She will probably tell you when she feels she needs more help with her medication'. We left each other with a much better understanding.

When I got back to the car, Joyce, another member of my staff, had left a message. The press had been on the phone asking what I thought about the doctor's repeat medication software that was printing the drug name for impotence instead of the one for smoking cessation. Would pharmacists know that it was the wrong drug on the prescription?

I telephoned the reporter back and explained that the mistake might be noticed when the patient was questioned about the use of the drug. All in all, a difficult situation for both the pharmacist and the patient. My particular comments were not used but I did read about an example of the problem the next day.

My third visit was to someone who was already taking his medicine from a compliance aid. Barny Hope had telephoned the pharmacy to say he didn't want any of his 'bone' medication sent until further notice. Barny had osteoporosis as well as diabetes and high blood pressure. It was easy to get into Mr Hope's house since there was a large notice on the door – 'Push the door – it's open!' I stepped over the umbrellas, walking sticks and wellingtons and made my way towards what looked like the lounge. 'Hello' I shouted, 'it's the pharmacist.'

The television was so loud that nothing could be heard. Obviously, from a safety point of view, Mr Hope was totally vulnerable. When I got myself into the lounge, I could just see the gentleman's head peering over a huge pile of newspapers. The gas fire was lit and I realised it would only take one of the papers to fall on the hearth, while Mr Hope slept, to create a fireball with tragic consequences. But first I needed to deal with the medication problems. I introduced myself but as I was still competing with the television, Mr Hope couldn't hear me. I searched around for the remote control and pressed the volume button firmly until he looked up, quite surprised to see me. He then asked who I was.

'Mr Hope, remember me, I telephoned earlier. It's the pharmacist about your medicines.' 'Oh yes – what's wrong again?' he said, looking a little puzzled. 'Mr Hope you need to keep taking your bone medicines to keep your bones strong. If you don't and you were to fall, you could break your leg and end up in hospital.'

I looked round the lounge and started to find lots of white boxes. One of the boxes contained the weekly medicine and the other the calcium and vitamin D tablets. Both are taken for osteoporosis and found to reduce the number of fractures in the over 65s. I had already counted twenty boxes when I headed into the bedroom and found another ten.

This was not working out. My staff would need to start putting the medication in the compliance aid despite the problems. One of the tablets has to be taken at a different time from any other medication and has to be taken at least half an hour before food. Mr Hope would need to make sure he remained upright after taking the medicine with a large glass of water. The calcium medication is uncoated and should generally be dispensed separately.

'So I'm going to put all your bone medicine in a separate tray but you need to take this one' – showing him one of the tablets out of the numerous white boxes – 'half an hour before food and at a different time from your other medication. It's only once a week. Can you take it with a large glass of water?' Mr Hope nodded and I headed for the door carrying all the extra medicine. He had more stock than my pharmacy!

Unfortunately, all of this medication would have to be destroyed since it cannot be reused. The health board has a contract with a waste disposal firm who uplift the pharmaceutical waste on a regular basis. This medicine waste adds up to hundreds of thousands of pounds every year.

Finally, I put the television volume up on the remote control, waved goodbye and headed for the door. I had noted the name of Mr Hope's carer and telephoned the agency when I got outside. I explained the unlocked door, the fire hazard and the medication problem and suggested they got in touch with the family. I explained I would also get in touch with them.

My final visit involved a lady, Jessie Whiteman, who had been discharged from hospital with a seven-day supply of her six different medicines all in similar looking white boxes. Her daughter, Karen, had phoned with a frantic message. 'I thought the surgery would automatically send you a prescription and Mrs Smith, my mother's friend, has a weekly tray. Can we have one as well because my mother is totally confused about when to take all her medicines?' This was all delivered in one breath and I could hear the panic in her voice.

This lady definitely needed help. She had had a stroke so I had to listen carefully as she answered my questions. I asked Karen for the discharge form from the hospital. When I was checking the new prescriptions with the form I noticed that one of the tablets had been missed. Her thyroxine tablets for her thyroid hadn't appeared on the new prescriptions, yet she had received a supply from the hospital.

I phoned Hilary again at the surgery and asked to speak to Dr Stephen this time. She said he was in surgery but would phone me back at the patient's house in between patients. I continued my checks with Mrs Whiteman and, after about five minutes, Dr Stephen phoned. Yes, she should continue with her thyroxine and he would issue a new prescription for tomorrow. Reflecting, I think it was about ten years earlier when I had written to the director of pharmacy at the Health board suggesting that community pharmacists should be sent a copy of the hospital discharge form for their patients since we could then check if first, the hospital had included all the 'old' drugs that had not been discontinued and that second, the surgery had included all the newly prescribed medication. We now have a service involving communication between hospital and community pharmacists that is proving very useful.

Now it was my turn to panic, or at least the girls back at the pharmacy. This lady was to have a weekly tray with all the paperwork delivered by the afternoon. I thought about my staff levels. Maybe if I asked Joyce or Trish to have a shorter lunch but get away earlier at night we could just about make it.

It was time to get back to the pharmacy and relieve my locum. Pharmacist owners need to employ locum pharmacists when they are out of the pharmacy in order to carry on the professional work.

I realised I would also need to deal with Dr Douglas's query before he started his surgery at three o'clock. As I approached the pharmacy, I was met by the lollipop man, Alex. I could see from his face that the news was not good. 'Did you know Jimmie Mitchell?' 'Yes', I answered knowing that something sombre was about to be uttered since he was using the past tense. 'Well', said Alex 'It was the last end in the match up at the green when he just keeled over. He couldn't finish the game and his team had to give away the cup.' 'Gosh', I said 'but I suppose it's a good way to go for him.' Alex agreed as he ushered me across the road. The parents of the children who used the crossing were always grateful for the care Alex took in keeping their charges safe.

As usual, the handover with the locum was quite lengthy since there had been several complications that morning. 'Mr Brown's dressings are unavailable from the manufacturer so I've left a message with the nurse prescriber.' Unfortunately, I thought, by the time the nurse gets back to us we will have probably missed the cut-off time for the next order. Louise, the locum looked down at the list she had written and continued, 'We've had a call from the Community Action Team saying that John will be bringing in a new prescription for an increased dose of his methadone so could we stop his present prescription?' Communication with us is paramount to avoid any doubling up of methadone doses.

'Mrs Grant's warfarin dose has to be changed.' I've annotated her notes. Mrs Grant is one of our 'weekly tray' ladies so I had visions of Joyce completely forgoing her lunch the way things were going. 'Oh I nearly forgot, a patient came in looking for some malaria tablets for Ethiopia. I'm afraid I haven't had time to look up the recommendation, sorry.'

I added that other query to my list. By this time I had waved goodbye to my own lunch and was about to tackle the pile of prescriptions that was waiting when the door opened and the inspector of our then regulatory body, the Pharmaceutical Society walked into the pharmacy. It reminds me a little of when you are stopped routinely by the police. You know you are innocent but there is always that feeling that something will be found that isn't quite correct.

He introduced himself and asked for the keys of the controlled drug cupboard. This is where we keep our 'morphine' type medicines and all paperwork must be 100% correct for both medicines received and dispensed. This was checked thoroughly and found to be accurate.

'Can I see your standard operating procedure paperwork and your private prescription book?' said the inspector. This is to check that members of staff are following safe procedures for all dispensing and the sale of medicines. The private prescription book is inspected for any irregular private prescriptions prescribed by doctors.

Thankfully, there were only some minor points regarding the procedures but the inspector's visit meant that my workload had been put on hold.

Closing time was looming and there was still a lot to do. Maybe I would have to stay late.

Yvonne came round the corner into the dispensary carrying a prescription with a worried look on her face. 'Mrs Grady says she's just got this prescription from the doctor but she doesn't want to take it.' This is a difficult situation because although it is up to the patient to make that decision, very often it is not in her best interest. I looked at the medicine that had been prescribed. It was for a hormone replacement therapy (HRT) preparation (which is given to try and lessen the symptoms of the menopause) so I went out to the front to deal with the situation. 'I've heard that these tablets can give you cancer' said Mrs Grady. 'There is a small increase in risk' I said 'but not enough to stop you trying the tablets out'. We had a quick discussion but the patient insisted she didn't want them and asked if there was an alternative medicine. At this point I told her if she was going down a separate route then I could help her but she would have to tell her doctor she was doing so. She agreed so I told her about some herbal remedies, lifestyle issues and particular foods to avoid. She left with the understanding that this was a trial and she should let her doctor know.

It was after half past six when I was putting the last padlock on the shutter when someone asked me 'Are you shut?' I wearily answered 'yes, but is there something you need?' 'Well it's my wee girl' the man said. 'She's got a bit of a temperature and we don't have any paracetamol in the house.' 'Sure' I said. 'I'll just open up and get you sorted' and so it was after 7pm when I got home!

Pharmaceutical care plans are now being integrated electronically into the modern pharmacy contract in 2013.

CHAPTER 2
SAVE THE SHOPS CAMPAIGN

Being in the community means getting involved with what's going on. Sometimes it means getting out of the pharmacy and taking part in community issues. I've always felt that the pharmacy is a bit like the post office. It needs to be at the heart of the community. If its status is threatened then I would be the first to challenge that decision.

Suddenly, the door burst open and John from the shop across the road came in and blurted out 'They're going to put bus lanes in Clarkston Road!' He reminded me a little of the character in 'Dad's Army': 'We're all doomed!'

Although I was making light of John's reaction the fact was, that if bus lanes were sited in Clarkston Road, then our businesses would suffer very badly indeed with some closures.

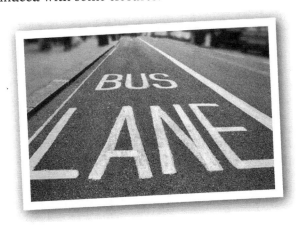

As I began to look at the situation, another couple of the local shopkeepers came in and suggested to me that fighting the roads department was no use. 'The council will always win' I heard several times. That was one of the reasons that I decided to rally the locals and put up a reasoned argument as to why this scheme shouldn't go ahead.

The first thing I did was ask the local councillor if he would like to help us and to start with, get me a venue to hold an action meeting. He agreed and the date was set for the following Thursday at the Couper Institute (the local hall). I printed out a batch of leaflets letting the local shopkeepers know about the meeting and asked them to please attend. I telephoned several key individuals for support and spent the next two nights traipsing up and down Clarkston Road slipping leaflets underneath shuttered shop doors after I finished work.

The Thursday of the meeting arrived and as usual I didn't get out on time from the pharmacy, so when I arrived at the Couper Institute and walked into the committee room, it was full of people not best pleased that I was late. I sat down at the top table beside the councillor expecting him to chair the meeting. Nothing was said so I quickly realised that I'd better say something, so I got the meeting started. A general discussion took place about whether a group of shopkeepers could actually overturn a decision made by the roads department but the main outcome was the agreement that we had to form a committee.

One of my friends, who had nothing to do with Clarkston Road but thought the campaign sounded fascinating, was charged with looking at the council's reasons for putting the bus lanes in place. These arguments included air pollution, numbers of cars and buses that used the route and congestion at the junctions along Clarkston Road at peak times. David was appointed secretary of the 'Save the Clarkston Road Shops' campaign and, as a retired scientist, he set to work with relish.

Mr McKnight from the bicycle shop was appointed treasurer and we agreed that if each shop paid £20 then we could use the funds for publicity. Mr Laurance Vallance from the carpet shop and Mr Perry from the gift shop were another two members of our committee and we started to decide our strategy and to plan the campaign.

The committee met for the first time the following week and our first question was – what could we do to raise our profile? We knew the best place to advertise our plight was going to be in the *Glasgow South and Eastwood Extra*, the local paper, so for that we needed stories. 'What about getting a coffin?' said Mat. We all looked at him wondering what he was thinking. He continued, 'We could get a coffin from the local funeral parlour and stop the traffic in Clarkston Road by walking in front of the coffin with 'Save the Clarkston Road Shops' banners and 'Stop the Bus Lanes' notices draped over it'.

'What a brilliant idea' I said and delegated the task of approaching the funeral director to the local councillor.

Our chosen day arrived, (thank goodness it was dry), and all of the committee, headed up by the councillor, started to walk up Clarkston Road just as we had planned. I began to wonder if I would be struck off as a pharmacist for taking part but I was pretty sure I would be exonerated when I told them why it had to be done. As we walked up the road, someone started shouting at the councillor, seemingly disagreeing with his political persuasion. It had nothing to do with our plight but it got us noticed. That stunt earned us a mention in the *Extra* newspaper.

The next publicity story was going to be with the help of the local circus. We went along to the park where the circus was being staged and the committee all climbed into a hot air balloon basket. We draped the appropriate banners on the basket and the caption in the paper was, 'Bus lanes in Clarkston Road are all about a lot of hot air.'

During the weeks of the campaign, we were constantly in touch with the roads department and at one point, went in to have a meeting about the proposal. The officials seemed very determined and astonished that we should think that this was not the best option for Clarkston Road. They told us about their plans to display the proposal in the Couper Institute in the library, for everyone to comment upon. I then asked them if they would be agreeable to coming along to an evening meeting that would be open to all members of the public.

The date was set for three weeks hence and I got everyone involved in giving out leaflets to all their customers urging them to help us fight the proposal. I appointed one person in each row of shops to go to their neighbours, explain the situation and ask for their help.

At the next committee meeting it was decided that we would have speakers from the shops who would make their points after the council representatives had made their case. I was to talk about the impact on businesses if the proposal went ahead. Laurance Vallance was going to raise the issue of general deterioration of the area as a result of the run-down shops and with a certainty of closures.

The meeting was to be held in the Couper Institute hall that held about 200 people. It was due to start at 7.30pm and at 7.25 there were five council officials and three committee members. My heart sank as I looked at the representatives' smug faces. Then something remarkable happened. At 7.28

pm some people started to arrive and by 7.32 pm there were at least 150 people in the audience.

The meeting started when the councillor stood up and introduced the road representatives. The first speaker from the department had an English accent. That would not normally be a problem except that he obviously hadn't done his homework and showed a complete lack of local knowledge. This resulted in some heckling from the audience and the chair had to calm the proceedings down before inviting our committee to speak.

We just spoke from the heart. What it would do to local businesses and the fact that there would be a rash of empty shops. The local economy would suffer and those who relied on the shops the most, such as the elderly and young families with no transport, would lose local services. At the question and answer session the local lollipop man Alex stood up and said, 'In all the 25 years I've been standing at the junction of Merrylee Road and Clarkston Road, I've never experienced a huge hold up.'

At this point the MP for the area, who was seated at the back of the hall, signalled to the representatives of the roads department to stop the proceedings. Remarkably, they seemed to have a statement ready and one of their number stood up and said, 'In view of the local opposition to the bus lanes plans, the roads department is dropping the case for bus lanes but would like to discuss other options to help the flow of traffic.'

We were ecstatic. We had won our case against all odds and there was much hugging and shaking of hands at our triumph. Several weeks later the department came back with sensible plans for some paid parking, disabled bays and clearway times. Yes, everyone on the committee and beyond had played their part. I was then invited to discuss our victory with the Victoria Road group, another south side team, but that's another story.

CHAPTER 3
MINOR AILMENTS

The minor ailments service in Scotland has been available in all community pharmacies since 2006. It means that children, people over 60, those with certain medical conditions, those on benefit and pregnant women (and for a year after birth) are eligible for the service. Many thousands of visits are made to pharmacies every day in Scotland. We act as the gatekeepers between the patient and the GP and can deal with many queries without having to visit the doctor. The service doesn't discriminate against people who are unable to pay for over-the-counter medicines. The pharmacist can then prescribe a medicine free of charge. In the 80s and 90s those people eligible for the service had to pay for an over-the-counter medicine. (In 2011, the Scottish Government abolished all prescription charges in Scotland).

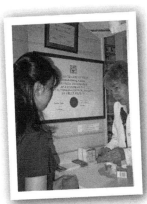

Counselling at the Semi-Private Area

The first example was far from minor.

Mrs White was gesticulating wildly from the back of the pharmacy, trying to catch my attention. She was an imposing woman with one of those distinctive voices that commanded action and, on this occasion, she urgently wanted to speak to me round at the semi-private area. I left the prescription I was dispensing in the capable hands of Linda, and headed round the corner. 'Do you think this is breast cancer?' she blurted out with desperation in her voice. I looked down at the exposed breast and the first thought that went though my head was 'Can anyone see this?' I wanted to protect this vulnerable woman. Luckily, no one else was within the vicinity so I turned my attention to answering the question. There was no obvious physical deformity so I told Mrs White that, first of all, most lumps found in the breast are not cancerous. I then told her the most important thing she should do is have an examination with her GP and I could organise that straightaway. I also noticed from her medication record that she was taking HRT (Hormone Replacement Therapy) and it would be important to stop the medication if breast cancer was diagnosed. (A thought I did not share with the patient.)

'Would you like me to make an appointment with your doctor for you?' With a trembling voice she thanked me and asked me to go ahead with the arrangement. Thankfully she was seen quickly, referred to the local hospital and was given a clear bill of health.

A rather harassed mother thrust a sticky piece of sellotape into my hand. Her two young children were pulling at her sleeve screeching 'Why are we in the chemist's and mummy can I have one of these?' Her younger daughter had picked up a packet of cough sweets and was unwrapping them in readiness to put them in her mouth. Vivian managed to rescue the sweets before any harm had been done.

I looked at the sellotape in my hand and realised it contained a head louse. Thankfully, the louse was dead and now I had to question – how many in the family were affected? 'They all are,' she said. With two young children snapping at her heels she was in no mood to answer questions but I had to emphasise the importance of only treating the children that had the infection. I continued my questioning and managed to ascertain that both children present had, after combing their hair, produced copious numbers of live lice.

I dealt with the lady quickly since I could see her children were becoming restless. I delegated the task of going over the directions with the mother to Trish as I saw there was another lady waiting with a query about her little girl.

'Do you think you could have a look at Amy's foot? I think it's a verruca.' I took the mother and daughter into the consulting room. 'Yes, it is a verruca' I confirmed so I want you to steep the foot in warm water for a few minutes and then dry carefully before applying this liquid.' As I was showing the mother the verruca preparation, the little girl piped up, 'Mummy, what's a steep?' I wanted to burst out laughing but managed to contain myself and gave a reasonable explanation. It was just another memorable moment.

I was about to see another patient when Yvonne gave me the phone - It's Dr Stephen for you.' 'Hello, how can I help you?' 'I just wanted to pass something by you,' said Dr Stephen. He continued, 'I want to change a patient to a diamorphine injection from oral morphine'. This is the sort of situation where I feel as if I am in a degree exam situation, knowing I have to think quickly on my feet. 'What's the total daily dose of morphine the patient is taking now?' I asked. With that information I was able to confirm Dr Stephen's calculation, say my goodbyes and ask Yvonne to send the next patient round.

He remained at the counter while shouting, 'I've got a skelf (splinter) stuck in my finger' as he brandished the offending object in front of Trish. I was fortunate to have employed a young medical student for the summer this particular year. Debbie completely took charge of the situation. It was like a real surgical operation in the consulting room. Wearing her surgical gloves, she used a sterile probe to prise the splinter out of the finger. The gentleman was over the moon and left the pharmacy regaling everyone with how marvellous we all were, since he had already visited the hospital with no success. Our medical student had performed the task impeccably.

I was dealing with a problem with an interaction with a new medicine that Linda had highlighted when she was dispensing Mr Maxwell's prescription when the man at the back of the pharmacy shouted, 'I've had enough I can't wait any longer!' and stormed out of the pharmacy. This is something with which all pharmacists have to contend. Because there is no appointment system, people come back in for prescriptions, emergencies happen and often someone who has asked to see the pharmacist is forgotten about.

Emergencies do happen. I was just about to check out Mr Black's itchy scalp in the consulting room when there was a shout from the door. 'Can the chemist come quick? An old lady has fallen outside the close and can't get up.' I grabbed my mobile phone (a rather large brick-like model at that time) excused myself from the waiting patient and rushed outside.

Pharmacists have got used to being summoned first when there's an accident. Yes, we are trained in first-aid but dealing with a serious accident can only be in a limited sense, for example taking charge of the situation and making sure the ambulance and police are called quickly.

When I looked up the road I realised it was Mrs Lewis, one of my 'weekly tray' patients. Two gentlemen had lifted her onto a seat that had miraculously appeared from the butcher's shop. (I knew that moving the patient after a fall is not the best thing to do but you just have to get on with things as they appear). 'Hello Mrs Lewis, it's the pharmacist here. Can you tell me if you feel any pain?'. I could see from where she was pointing she had probably broken her hip so I asked the assembled crowd if anyone had phoned for an ambulance. 'No, we were waiting for you' said one of the men that had lifted Mrs Lewis up. I reached into my white coat pocket for my phone and dialed 999. I was explaining the situation to the operator when Mrs Lewis shouted, 'I'm not going to hospital!' I finished my report to the ambulance service, hung up and turned back to the patient. It was absolutely imperative that she was admitted to hospital so I knew I had to try my best counselling skills. 'Mrs Lewis,' I said, 'how are you going to prepare your food or go to the toilet if you can't stand?' 'I'll manage' she retorted, but I could hear her resolve was beginning to falter. By this time the paramedics had arrived but because Mrs Lewis was being so unco-operative, the ambulance crew were going to leave empty-handed. I made one last stab at persuading her to get into the ambulance by saying I was about to phone her daughter who would be very angry to hear she hadn't gone to hospital.

That did it. She was lifted into the back of the ambulance and, after returning the chair to the butcher's shop, I headed back to John Black's scalp. The gentleman was still waiting patiently in the consulting room. Having asked a few questions about how long he had the itch and how it felt, I donned a pair of surgical gloves and had a look at his scalp. 'Mmmm' I said 'it looks like shingles.' 'What does that mean?' said Mr Black. 'Well, shingles is a rather nasty viral infection and you want to get it treated as soon as possible to avoid nerve pain in the future. Look I'll try and catch the doctor who will want to have a look at the rash. If he agrees then we'll get you started on a course of medication.' A quick phone call had John over at the surgery within the hour. One of the GPs wrote a prescription and the patient got started on the tablets that evening. 'Remember, take the tablets five times a day, four hours between and for five days.' I could see John was a bit puzzled so I drew five clock faces on a piece of paper. 'These are the times you want to take the medication. Please take them as prescribed. We know that if you do, it could avoid the pain lingering on.' 'Thanks a lot Mrs Roddick,' Mr Black said as he headed out the door.

Then it happened. How did it happen? The Mr Smith of Steele Road was in for his prescription but it was not there. On the other hand, another prescription for a second Mr Smith at a completely different address was still in the pharmacy. I remember I had stated the address to the first patient and he had nodded and picked up the prescription. The protocol in the pharmacy is always to ask the patient the address since some people can mishear or simply not listen to a member of staff. My stomach was rapidly sinking into my gut and my heart was beating rapidly. I needed to take control quickly.

I directed Linda to re-dispense the prescription for the Mr Smith who was standing waiting in the pharmacy. I then tried to find the phone number of the first Mr Smith but as usual, when it's needed urgently, I found it was ex-directory. The receptionist at the surgery promised to phone the patient and ask him to get in touch with the pharmacy as soon as possible.

After what seemed an age, it was in fact only about twenty minutes, the phone rang. 'Yes, hello Mr Smith thank you for getting in touch. Basically, I have mistakenly given you another patient's prescription. I am very sorry that this has happened. Have you started to use the cream?' 'No' he answered. I continued, 'Can I ask you to call back into the pharmacy? If it's not convenient, I can get a member of staff to deliver your prescription to your home.' Mr Smith said he would call in shortly and with a huge sigh of relief the emergency was over. The incident was certainly not over as far as the pharmacy was concerned. Any critical incident, which this was, has to be looked at carefully. How did it happen and what safeguards have to be put in place? The essential outcome is that this incident must never happen again and so from this, we learned that asking the patient for the address is mandatory.

So, the afternoon moved on and several people arrived in with various degrees of viral infections. My staff were all checking how long they had had the problem, was there something worrying about symptoms and whether they were on any medication before deciding to refer to the GP or suggest some remedy.

It was at this point when a gentleman arrived carrying a prescription. His demeanour was a mixture of exasperation, anger and anxiety. I asked him if I could help. He explained that he had been round several pharmacies but couldn't get the prescription dispensed. I checked the name of the medicine on his prescription and realised that this was a drug for prostate cancer. I could understand his anxiety but I knew that this particular medication was unavailable from the manufacturer.

'I'll tell you what I suggest, there are a couple of makes of the same medication that you require. Tomorrow, I'll phone your GP and ask for another make of the drug and get it ordered for you for the afternoon.' The gentleman was just so grateful it lifted the whole mood of the pharmacy.

We were getting near closing time when a man came in asking for a very strong painkiller. 'It's for my wife. She's got a headache and nothing seems to be working.' By this time alarm bells were ringing in my ears. Was there any history of headaches? The man thought for a minute then said he remembered his wife had had an arterial headache – 'Is that the right name?' he asked. 'Listen,' I said. My tone had changed. 'Can you take your wife down to the out-of-hours department right now? I'll give you a referral letter.' He agreed and left.

We were just closing up when he reappeared with a prescription for steroids. This lady had a type of migraine that could lead to blindness if not treated quickly with steroids. She had been very lucky.

I thought the day was over when my husband and I arrived home after a meal out with friends. It was just after midnight when the phone went. 'Hello, this is Dr.Forbes from the Victoria out-of-hours department. I have a patient in the last few hours of life. She needs some palliative care medication'.

We are called a palliative care pharmacy and that means we carry all the medication needed for seriously ill patients at the end of life. Dr Forbes continued, asking for a list of medications and we agreed to meet at the pharmacy so that I could take a look at the prescription. There are legal requirements concerning how the prescriptions are written, so it is much easier to sort out any discrepancies with the doctor in front of me.

It was 12.45am when I labelled all the drugs required in the pharmacy. There was a complication, however. I didn't have one of the drugs in stock so the only thing I could think of doing was to a call another colleague out and meet her at her pharmacy. To get her home number I had to go through the emergency out-of-hours telephone system first. I met the other pharmacist at her pharmacy half an hour later. We must have looked respectable as we opened up in the early hours of the morning since two police officers were sitting in a patrol car a few yards away, quite relaxed.

Time was marching on when I finally got all the medication together. I then had to deliver it to an area I didn't know. I telephoned out-of-hours and asked the nurse if she could look at a street map and talk me through the directions. (We didn't have SatNav then). I had to stop the car a couple of times to phone in to check where I was going. It was about half past one when I got to the lady's door. The nurse was very grateful when I handed over the package but I had to go back again to my car to get the prescriptions. I had forgotten to get her signature on the back of them for receipt of the controlled drugs. What a night!

CHAPTER 4
THE METHADONE SERVICE

The methadone supervision programme started in the 90s when a few enlightened pharmacists in Glasgow realised that, if the patient was to take the dose in the pharmacy, then that would reduce methadone ending up on the streets. Officials at the health board, GPs and pharmacists then started to work together to try and deal with the growing drug problem and ultimately save lives. The justice system was in favour of the service since methadone stabilises patients, meaning they generally don't need to steal or cause criminal damage for illicit drugs.

There are some people who remain on methadone for years but it can allow many of them to get back into society. Getting extra training and a job can mean they can lead a 'normal' life where methadone fits round that.

But what is unique about the programme is the fact that community pharmacists end up with a special relationship with this group of patients. We see them daily and get involved in their lives, both the good parts and the bad.

I first found out about Sharon when she was weaving her way dangerously in between traffic and was carrying what looked like a silver cup. She was hotly pursued by Father McKinnon from the church who, in a past life, had been a professional rugby player. So, when he made his final tackle and Sally lay prostrate on the pavement, it looked quite spectacular. By this time, a crowd had gathered on Langside Drive and someone had phoned the police. It wasn't long, with sirens blazing before Sharon was picked up (literally) by two policemen and was whisked away in their van.

Not long after that, Sharon came into the pharmacy to ask if I was willing to take her onto the methadone programme. Pharmacists have to decide on the numbers of patients that they can comfortably handle within the normal pharmacy business. Methadone patients sometimes require time and can be difficult to deal with if doses are missed and we have to refuse to give them their medication.

So I had a free slot for Sharon and I signed her up by getting her to fill in the pharmacy contract. This is a contract between the methadone patient and the pharmacy. It sets out the expected standards of behaviour, the preferred times for the patients to come for their methadone, and what will happen if daily doses are missed.

She told me she had moved from Manchester and, after a period of homelessness, had met her current partner and they had settled in Glasgow. They were living in a flat in the area.

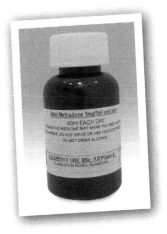

A Methadone Dose

Sharon saw from the contract that she had to wait until her name was called to come round to the consultation area. Because this semi-private area was used for all patients, there was no stigma attached to the fact that they were taking their methadone behind the screen.

After drinking a small amount of water and speaking to me – ensuring no methadone is retained in the mouth – Sharon left . Sharon was a model patient. She always arrived on time, sat down and waited until her name was called and after taking her dose, quietly left the pharmacy.

This particular day, she looked quite agitated and when I called her over she suddenly started to sob uncontrollably. I wanted to get her into the consulting room but there was a problem. There were podiatry instruments in the room. Normally, I would trust Sharon but in her distressed state, she would have to be chaperoned. Trish went with her and I went back to the dispensary to get Sharon's methadone dose. I realised that I would have to get Sharon out of the room quickly since I was tying up a member of staff and the prescriptions were piling up.

Amazingly, Clair my emergency locum walked into the pharmacy. 'I've just dropped off my grandchild at the school and I thought I'd come in and get my own prescription,' she said. I could have hugged her. 'Clair,' I said excitedly, 'can you do a locum for an hour while I sort out a problem?' 'Yes' said Clair 'but I've got my keep fit class at 11.'

Pharmacists such as Clair are a godsend. How does a full time pharmacist get to the dentist, the bank or the hairdresser? I also find pharmacists that can just come in for a short time means patients can be booked in for a consultation without disrupting the flow of the pharmacy business.

That meant I could relieve Trish in the room. 'Sharon, what's going on?' Still speaking through tears she started 'He's only f......... coming up to Glasgow! Oh, sorry for swearing' (That's not allowed in the contract). 'Who is?' I asked. 'My father.' She spat out the words. 'I ran away when I was sixteen. I couldn't stand it. I didn't tell him where I'd gone.' Sharon started to tell me about her home life and I began to put two and two together realising that she had been abused by her father as she grew up in her home in Manchester. 'It was when I was on the streets when this guy gave me some drugs. He showed me a way out and I came to Glasgow. I never told my family where I moved. I don't understand it. Who told him?'

I didn't have an answer but the fact that she was starting to talk calmed her down and eventually she was ready to leave. Telling the story of her earlier life seemed to change the relationship between us so when she appeared another day again in tears I assumed there had been a meeting with her father. No, not this time.

'I'm pregnant' she wailed. 'What will happen to the baby?' Sharon seemed genuinely upset about her first pregnancy so I said I would find out from the specialist pharmacist at the health board what was best for her and the baby.

The pharmacist suggested Sharon should try reducing her methadone dose so I told her to speak to her GP and that I would support her through the nine months. The baby growing inside her changed her outlook and she became focussed on doing what she thought was best.

Eight and a half months later Sharon rushed into the pharmacy and cried out 'My waters broke!' That was when the panic started. I certainly didn't want Sharon to have her baby in the pharmacy so I shouted. 'Where's your partner?' 'He's outside in the car.' 'Yvonne, I need you to go outside and get Pete in here as quickly as possible. Tell him he'll need to take Sharon to the hospital.' It seemed a split second later when Pete came rushing into the pharmacy. 'What's happening?' he exclaimed waving his arms about like a demented hyena. 'You've got to get Sharon to the Southern General now – she's about to have your baby!' 'Where is the f........... Southern General?' he shouted frantically. 'Do you know where Ibrox is?' 'Yeah' – he knew where his team played. 'Well get to Ibrox and turn left. Follow the signs for the hospital.' Pete dragged Sharon out the door and they were gone. Two weeks later, Sharon came in with her new baby boy, Rob, and that was the last time I saw her.

Ian came in for his dose as usual but this time he was weaving about the front shop obviously intoxicated. It's quite clear in the contract that if anyone is the worse for wear with alcohol then the dose of methadone is refused. I called him over to the window. 'Ian you know the rules' I started. 'You f........ b...... give me my methadone.' That was enough. 'If you don't calm down I'll have to call the police.' That seemed to have an impact because his demeanour changed. 'Tell you what Ian, I'm going to phone your community worker and, if you go away and sober up and come back just before closing we'll see what we can do.' Thankfully, that worked and Ian headed out the door.

Suzanne was booked up to work in Singapore. There was, however, a problem. She was on methadone and clearly Singapore and drugs do not work. She embarked on a programme of reducing her dose steadily over a period of time. It was very important she stuck to the regime because of her ultimate goal – the lure of a new life in an exciting city far away from her earlier traumatic lifestyle. The dose was reduced over a period of four months until ultimately, she was only taking 1ml daily. (That's about a fifth of a teaspoon.)

At this stage, it seemed like a psychological crutch. The presenting daily at the pharmacy, the discipline of this activity meant that she was determined to succeed. Finally the day came when she no longer used methadone in her life. Two weeks later she called in to tell us that she was catching her plane the next day and I think it was about six months later when we received a postcard saying that she was enjoying her new job and particularly her new life. Will Suzanne ever go back to her addiction? I hope not.

There are tragedies as well as success stories. Colin was one of those fresh-faced youths with an engaging smile. He was taking 50ml of methadone but was determined to come off it. He had a part-time job as a joiner and wanted to make it full time. 'As soon as I am straight,' he said. We embarked on a set reduction routine where Colin's GP lowered his dose every fortnight.

He was off methadone exactly as he said he would be. I have never seen someone so elated, so full of life with an expectation for a new start. I shook his hand and wished him well.

It was several weeks later when the police arrived in the pharmacy to question me on the last time Colin received a dose of methadone, I realised something was wrong. Colin had taken an over-dose at a party the Saturday before. He was dead.

Perhaps methadone isn't the answer long term, but for now, it's one way of tackling the increase in il-licit drug use in society. I certainly will never forget that part of my service.

CHAPTER 5
CHRISTMAS DAY OPENING

Community pharmacies all over the UK are open during public holidays to make sure that the public gets the medication and advice they need.

This was one Christmas I won't forget.

It was October 2000 and Joyce told me that Janine from the health board was on the phone. 'Hello Janine, how can I help you?'

'I wondered if your pharmacy could open on Christmas and New Year's Day for three hours?' she replied. My first thoughts were what would my husband and I be doing on those days and how would he feel if I was working? 'Well he is so used to my working then I suppose it won't make too much difference', I inwardly thought. 'Yes' I replied 'but I will need to check with my staff first. I'll let you know tomorrow.' I hung up and thought about the different members of staff. I would probably start by asking the students since, with no family commitments and the promise of double wages, I thought I could persuade at least two of them to volunteer.

And that's exactly what happened so, on Christmas Day, I rounded the corner approaching the pharmacy to find to my astonishment a long queue of people standing waiting for me to open up. There were all ages – from a tiny baby in arms to a very elderly gentleman who shouldn't have been out on that very frosty morning. I knew from the workload the previous week and from all the news items on television and in newspapers that we were seeing a huge increase in patients with flu-like symptoms.

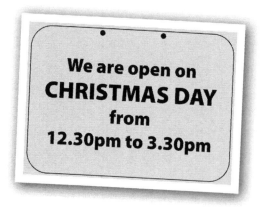

We are open on
CHRISTMAS DAY
from
12.30pm to 3.30pm

Opening up the pharmacy I felt a slight degree of panic. There were a lot of anxious people depending on us and I knew we would have to deliver a first-class service to get through the work. As soon as I got into the pharmacy, the phone started ringing and the first query was, 'Where is your pharmacy?' I was obviously the only pharmacy open and people were coming from miles around.

On realising that the phone calls on directions were going to be problematic since neither myself nor my staff would have time to spend on directing people, I telephoned my mother and asked if she would 'man' the phone. Obviously, if it was a medical query, then I would take over I told her. In the year 2000 my mother was 84 years old and only had about 1% vision. She had, however, driven in Glasgow all her adult life and had an amazing memory for street names.

My two members of staff arrived and started to deal with the massive crowd who were now jostling for a place at the counter. One woman shouted 'It won't take long will it – it's only tablets?' I could see Derek ready to retaliate and I remembered a story my father had told me about his colleague faced with the same comment. This elderly pharmacist had turned round and, lifting a bottle of bile beans, (a laxative), placed it directly on the lady's prescription. 'There you are' he said looking directly at her. The woman retorted 'These aren't my tablets' to which he replied, 'Well you said it was only tablets, so that's what I've given you.'

I never heard how that scene ended but I always hoped that people would understand the complexities of medicines and why we need to be professionally qualified to supply drugs to the public.

The phone was going about every five minutes and I could hear my mother handling all the queries very well until she called me over. Someone was needing help with her father-in-law. 'He's dropped all his medicine on the bed out of his weekly dispenser that we made up for him. They don't know his sleeping tablets from his water ones what should they do?'

'Can you bring them all down to the pharmacy and I will try and sort them out?' I said.

At that point I was able to hand the phone back to my mother who had to tell the Irish daughter-in-law where we were. Once again, my mother came up trumps.

I looked at the pile of prescriptions on the bench and the crowd of people that seemed to be getting larger and realised that I would have to phone another member of staff to see if they could come in.

'Hello is that Mark?' 'Hello Mrs Roddick, merry Christmas,' he answered, 'I'm just enjoying the view from the George the Fifth bridge on this crisp sunny morning.'

'Well' I said 'never mind the view, can you get in here pronto, I've never seen so many people in my life, we can't cope!'

Mark managed to get to the pharmacy in twenty minutes and went straight to work on the growing prescription queue in a systematic manner. One of the doctors who had just come on duty at the out-of-hours centre was prescribing an antibiotic that we never used in the community. I got hold of one of the out-of-hour nurses and told her what we did have in stock and so, after a discussion with the doctor, he changed his prescribing. That stopped a lot of delays with having to change prescriptions after speaking to the prescribing doctors.

At this point, there was a bit of a rumpus. One of the prescriptions had got out of order and someone had inadvertently skipped the queue. I think it is called a 'herd' reaction where one person started to complain about not getting their prescription on time and that sentiment started to spread through the crowd until the anger could be felt wafting into the dispensary. I haven't often been frightened in my working life but I felt threatened by the mounting aggression. The only thing we could do was to keep our heads down, speak civilly to everyone and work as quickly as possible.

The phone rang again, and this time it was a lady shouting about the fact that we had never picked up her prescription from the surgery. I called over to Mark and said we couldn't do anything because of the holiday but we would sort it out as soon as the doctors were back. At that point she shouted, 'Don't bother I'll get it from another pharmacy!' and slammed the phone down. I often wondered if patients ever spoke to their doctors like that or was it just pharmacists and pharmacies that seemed to sometimes bear the brunt of the angry patient? Ninety-nine per cent of my regular customers and patients were so pleasant and a delight to deal with, so I held onto that thought as we battled through the day.

This particular flu had symptoms of a rather nasty cough and a high temperature so everyone was buying paracetamol and a cough bottle as well as getting their prescription. Very soon it became apparent that we were going to run out of over-the-counter medicines. What could I do? Yes, of course, borrow from a colleague on the other side of town.

This is where my husband came in. 'Hello Douglas – yes I know you're in the middle of cooking the turkey but can you go over to Paisley Road West and borrow six dozen paracetamol and the same of pholcodine linctus (a cough bottle) and I'll phone Alasdair the pharmacist and let him know?'

My husband arrived in the pharmacy with the extra stock within half an hour. It was like Armageddon, with people jostling to purchase what they needed for their families.

An older lady came round to collect the prescription for her husband. The medication ordered was for a morphine type of medicine. The lady obviously wanted to talk so I asked her who the prescription was for. 'It's John, my husband,' she said. He had been diagnosed with cancer a few months back but he was now needing a strong painkiller. I placed my hand over hers, words didn't seem right at that moment. She smiled at me with a tear in her eye and left. She continued to come back into the pharmacy for many months after that until the inevitable happened. Building relationships and helping people in time of need is what I love about my work. Being there for families when a loved one is at the end of life is probably the most important time to make sure that we have all the medication needed and are able to get that to the patient quickly.

The elderly gentleman who had been in the queue asked if he could speak to me and, when I took him round to the consultation area, he explained that he was worried about his wife. She was also in her eighties and with the description he was giving me it sounded like shingles that needed to be treated quickly. I made the mistake of phoning out of hours and giving the patient's wrong date of birth since that had been transcribed wrongly onto a repeat prescription slip. The upshot was no-one was willing to speak to me and I had to send the gentleman home to phone himself to ask for a doctor to call. Thankfully now there is a complete communication channel between pharmacies open on Saturdays and public holidays with the out-of-hours services.

I thought we were getting through the work quite well when a quite extraordinary thing happened. The door burst open and a young man, flanked by two police officers, came into the pharmacy and made his way towards the counter. I could see that the young man was handcuffed to both officers but he looked like any well-groomed twenty year-old. His shirt was clean and recently pressed while his trousers were well cut and expensive. He was the sort of young man that any mother would have been proud of, yet here he was shackled to two policeman and present in the pharmacy to get a dose of methadone.

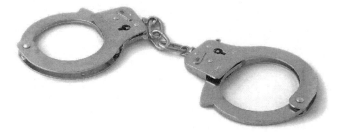

When it was his turn to receive his prescription, I called his first name – Christopher – and the three men moved as one into the consultation area. One of the policemen unlocked the handcuffs so that Christopher could take his dose and for the first time he lifted his head and looked directly at me. I could see from his eyes he was sorry. He didn't have that defiant look that many of the young men that get into trouble have. He looked humiliated. After the mandatory drink of water I spoke to him and he thanked me. Not having to take his methadone in front of all the other patients had obviously helped him retain some self-esteem, even for a moment.

By this time we were starting to get to the end of the prescriptions but there were several people in looking to have a word about some annoying medical complaint that hadn't merited calling the doctor. There was the child with a flare-up of eczema who just needed an effective moisturiser to help calm things down over the next couple of days and the gentleman who had hurt his back putting up Christmas decorations the night before. He was given some anti-inflammatories and a heat-rub with the express instructions to take the tablets after food and see his doctor after the holidays if things hadn't improved.

Finally, the last patient had left. We all looked at each other in silent awe. Somehow we had managed to cope with the vast number of patients and what that meant for our pharmacy. Yes we could now go home and enjoy our Christmas dinners with our families knowing that we had tried our best to give a good service that day.

CHAPTER 6
EMERGENCY HORMONAL
CONTRACEPTIVE SERVICE

The young boy nervously approached the counter. 'Could I speak to the pharmacist?' he said in a faltering voice. Linda ushered him round to the consultation area and when he approached me he looked terrified. His voice was almost inaudible when he asked me if he could get the morning-after pill. I looked at his frightened face and carefully and quietly explained he would need to bring his girlfriend in so that I could have a word with her. 'She won't come in. She's too scared' he said. 'Tell her that everything is treated confidentially and tell her that it would be best if she came in and had a chat,' I explained.

The boy disappeared and I hadn't expected him to reappear but, sure enough, about half an hour later he came in with a young girl with a shock of red hair hiding her face. She was obviously very upset. 'Come into the consultation room and have a seat,' I said.

I'm never sure whether the partner is invited to come in as well and in this case she wanted to be on her own. There are a series of questions that are asked to make sure that no more than 72 hours have elapsed since the unprotected sex and also, whether it was possible, within the cycle, that a pregnancy could already have occurred. She was close to crying as she answered the questions. This was obviously not a young girl who was using the 'morning-after' pill for contraception as some young girls do. When I got to the questions on medical conditions and whether she was on any medication both from her doctor and also over-the-counter she was sobbing and I had to stop for a few minutes while she composed herself. 'Yes' she faltered 'I'm on St John's Wort'. This is an herbal remedy for mild depression and normally it wouldn't be a problem but in this case it was. 'The St John's Wort,' I explained, 'will interfere with the contraceptive so you will have to take double the dose'. I thought to myself – this is outside the licensing indications. I'm going to have to phone out-of-hours. 'Could you excuse me? I'll be back in a minute.'

Back in the dispensary Trish was trying to attract my attention. 'What's wrong?' I said. 'Shhhh,' she put her finger to her lips. 'This looks like a dodgy prescription.' She pointed to the handwritten form in front of me that was for gliclazide (a diabetic drug), lactulose (a laxative) and temazepam (a sleeping tablet with a high street value). I thought to myself, thank goodness for well-trained staff, from the medicine counter assistants right through to the dispensers and dispensing technicians. They have all gone through rigorous training in order to contribute to the safe running of the pharmacy.

Here was a case in point. It was Trish that had brought this to my attention.

'Yes it looks like a forged prescription' I said in a hushed voice. 'Is it going to be long?' the young man shouted over into the dispensary. 'It'll just be a few minutes – why don't you have a seat?' I shouted back. Obviously, if he had been a seasoned forger, then he would be looking for signs of our spotting the forgery and would be ready to run. I took the phone into the back and called the surgery that had produced the prescription. No, they didn't have a patient with that name and address and Dr Wilson's pad had been stolen that morning said the receptionist. I thanked her and told her I was going to phone the police. This is always a tricky situation because the forger standing in the pharmacy could suddenly turn violent and someone could get hurt. Speed was of the essence. I dialled 999 and explained who I was and what was happening.

We had all been taught to carefully but discreetly observe the individual so we could give detailed descriptions to the police. The young man was wearing a brown leather jacket. He had unkempt long brown hair and was overweight. I'd managed to alert Linda in the front and so, when he handed her an empty can of coke, she knew that this would be evidence if the man had been caught. He seemed to get quite anxious because of the time it was taking to dispense the prescription and suddenly turned and marched out of the pharmacy. Unfortunately the police didn't arrive for some time so they only had our descriptions, an empty can of coke, plus a vague direction as to where he was headed. We never heard whether he had been caught.

Fifteen minutes had elapsed and I realised that the young woman was still in the consulting room. I entered the room, apologised about the delay and explained that I was going to phone out-of-hours to ask if they could see her quickly.

'Yes', said the nurse, the doctor could see her if she came down now and she would give the girl a prescription for the two EHC (Emergency Hormonal Contraceptive) tablets. The girl and her boyfriend left for the hospital. They returned in an hour with the prescription and we were able to dispense it quickly. There was no charge for the NHS prescription but if the girl had had to pay without a prescription, it would have been around £20.

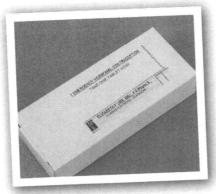

Emergency Hormonal Contraception

In 2013, this service is now part of the community pharmacy contract in Scotland and free of charge.

At this point, I received a call from an elderly lady who had just taken a dose of penicillin and had come out in a nasty rash. She wondered what she should do. 'Don't take any more of your tablets and I'll come up with an antihistamine for you as soon as I have finished here'. I checked her medication record on the computer to find out if there was any problem with her taking an antihistamine as well. I then labelled a packet ready to take with me.

When I arrived at the lady's house she showed me the extensive rash and, making sure there were no other worrying symptoms, I told her to take one tablet now and one going to bed. 'It is also important to let your doctor know in the morning about what's happened so that he can mark it in your surgery notes and maybe prescribe another antibiotic if necessary.' I then headed out the door. The next day, I telephoned the company that had manufactured the antibiotic and asked for a printout of all the ingredients in their formulation. I then sent that information to her GP. The last thing I did was fill in a Yellow Card [6] about the adverse reaction relating to the lady's rash. The card is sent away and the information is pooled centrally so that checks can be kept on medicine safety. It used to be only the medical profession that could fill in a card but now, in 2013, anyone, including members of the public, should report any problem including herbal remedies and supplements.

CHAPTER 7
TALKING WITH GPs

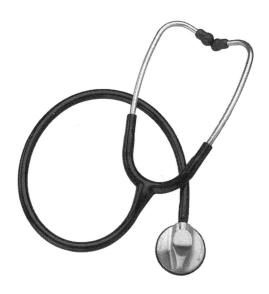

In the 1980s and early 90s communication with GPs was very limited. In my own practice, I wanted to try and change that if I could.

'What have I done this time?' said Uncle Douglas in a half serious and half jovial mood. Uncle Douglas was the affectionate name everyone called the senior partner at the local practice. 'Well it's just to check a dose for child – Amy McKinnon aged seven,' I replied.

It did seem that I was on the phone at least twenty times a day for sometimes trivial things such as changes in pack sizes of medicines or a patient had moved address so did they want to change their computer system as well? Sometimes it was about an interaction with a medicine or maybe just a dose check. So I decided to ask the doctors if it would be better if I came to the surgery once a month with a pile of non-urgent prescriptions to be changed and to get them all done at once.

When the senior partner retired, it was ultimately Dr McKay who took over the task. 'Hello Kathleen, can you check when Dr McKay will be available for the 'homework' next week?' That's what I called the pile of prescriptions that had to be altered. 'Yes,' said Kathleen, 'I can give you a slot next Wednesday at 12.30pm.'

To make the whole process as time-efficient as possible I would fax over a list of names and addresses of patients whose prescriptions needed altering and one of the receptionists would type out the 'appointments' so each patient's computer record could be accessed quickly. At the exact time agreed, I would appear at the surgery. 'Hello Dr McKay – quite a large list today.' 'So I see, so let's get started.'

Dr McKay was a very efficient doctor and we rattled through the list quickly. This meeting also gave me the chance to bring up some pharmacy news such as a change in legislation regarding prescribing a particular drug, or that a product was being discontinued. I felt that having a locum in for an hour to allow me to 'do' the homework was well worth the expense and the time saved on both the doctor's and the pharmacy side. There were very few 'What have I done now?' moments after that.

During the early 90s, GPs were being appointed by the Scottish Office as prescribing advisors. It soon became apparent that what was required were pharmacists to work with the advisors and Greater Glasgow Health Board appointed two pharmacists to that position, Margaret Mackie and Angela Timoney. Clare Mackie, community pharmacist, led the way developing individual pharmaceutical care plans for patients while working in GP practices.

In 1991, at a training event in Edinburgh, I heard a talk from a hospital pharmacist who had gone into some GP practices to give a presentation about prescribing. I came away from that meeting full of ideas and I thought maybe, just maybe, I could do the same with my local GPs

I learned early on that it's much better to ask for help with a project like this. I had heard there was some Scottish Office funding and, with the help from the Pharmaceutical General Council, the body that used to negotiate with government on fees for community pharmacists, I managed to obtain a grant.

Elspeth, Carol and Colin from the organisation were instrumental in helping put the project together and submitting it for publication. Up-to-date medicine information would be key to the success of the research so I contacted the information pharmacist at the Victoria Infirmary.

'Hello Kate, would you be able to help me with research papers on the different topics, and then listen to my talks on prescribing, before I go into the GP surgeries?' Kate sounded intrigued. 'Yes, tell me what you need and we'll see what we can do.' What I wanted to do with my research was to see if, after I gave my talk to the GPs on each topic, their prescribing changed.

I wrote to each GP practice in the area explaining about the Scottish Office grant and whether they would be willing to take part by listening to four, half-hour lunchtime talks about prescribing. Amazingly, they all agreed but I did find a real challenge at the beginning. They weren't used to someone questioning their prescribing. They also had to give me permission to look at their health board data to see if my talks had altered prescribing in any way. I couldn't believe how nervous I was at the first talk I did. I had practised it in front of two information pharmacists for accuracy but also in front of my husband.

'Are there any questions?' I asked my husband at the end of the talk. 'Yes' he said 'why are you wearing that ridiculous top?' I scolded him for not understanding my anxiety but he then made the right noises like, 'Yes, it sounds OK but I don't know what you're talking about!'

The first talk loomed. I was ushered into the largest consulting room and noticed that one of the partners was still signing repeat prescriptions and obviously not listening to what I was saying. 'Who is this woman wasting our time?' she was probably thinking. Ironically, it was this doctor that used to phone me with questions at least twice a day after I had finished the four talks.

In another practice, I decided to just give the talk to one of the partners so I could compare the prescription data of the other two GPs. In this case, I was squeezed into a tiny consulting room just before the surgery started so things were quite tense. Despite the fact that patients were starting to arrive in the waiting room just outside, I managed to get the salient points across. The depth of the GP's questions proved to me that he was interested in my information.

The third practice seemed at the time to be the most civilised. I was invited for lunch where we chatted generally about the NHS, patients and resources. After that, I gave my talk to a relaxed ensemble that tested my knowledge with taxing questions. One of the GPs was going to be one of the advisors already mentioned to help her colleagues prescribing within another health board and we ended up working together on newsletters about best practice.

When I collected all my data, I then put a questionnaire to the GPs. Were the talks useful? 'Yes', for the most part with comments such as, 'Interesting, informative and unbiased' and, 'More balanced than drug reps' talk.'

I also decided to put a rather cheeky question to them. 'How would you feel if doctors diagnosed and pharmacists prescribed?' In 1991, certainly with the older doctors, it was a bridge too far but the younger ones felt, if the pharmacist had all the necessary information about the patient, they didn't see that as a problem.

'There is a gentleman on the phone from the College of Pharmacy Practice in Warwick,' said Joyce as she handed me the phone. 'Yes', I said, 'Elizabeth Roddick here.' 'Congratulations' the gentleman on the other end of the phone said, 'you have won the Schering Award for your pioneering work talking to GPs about their prescribing'. I was flabbergasted but also elated since the research had taken over my life for two years and when it was published in the Pharmaceutical Journal [4], I thought that had been the ultimate prize. But to receive this award mainly because one of the GPs had put in a written submission about how helpful the talks had been was the real icing on the cake.

The managing director of Schering, the pharmaceutical company that awarded the prize, visited my pharmacy shortly after that. He then wrote a letter in the Pharmaceutical Journal about his experience called 'A life in the day of' [5] where he expresses his surprise at the work done in a pharmacy and also the impact that his industry can have on patient care. An example was one of his company's drugs arriving into the pharmacy with the bottle smashed and the resultant delay for the patient.

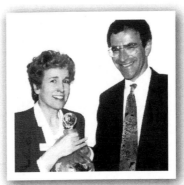

Mike Wallace Schering Managing Director
Presenting The Award

Later, Glasgow led the way with pharmacists producing individual care plans for patients by working within GP practices. In 2013, there is an army of pharmacists employed by health boards and health authorities going into surgeries helping with cost-effective prescribing.

What could I do next? Yes I was going to become an independent prescriber. That required going back to university with essays, exams and mentoring by one of the local GPs, Dr McKay.

I held my first clinic on osteoporosis in 2001.

Mrs McKeeve had been to the Southern General for a bone scan and now her results were back. I stood up when the patient entered the room. 'How do you do Mrs McKeeve, my name is Elizabeth Roddick and I'm going to have a discussion with you about your results from the hospital.'

Mrs McKeeve was slightly taken aback and immediately asked if Dr Douglas was going to see her as well. I then explained that, with all the results now available, I would be prescribing the new medication for her condition. The receptionist had told the patients that I would be holding the clinic but Mrs McKeeve hadn't picked that up. She settled down and I went through the different medicines I was prescribing for her and emphasised how important it was to continue taking the medicines to prevent any further breaks.

'Are there any side effects?' Mrs McKeeve replied. 'Is there not something to do with an effect on your teeth with one of them?' Interestingly enough, that was one of the questions I had asked the consultant at the Southern General. (Part of my course had meant spending time with a consultant who saw the more difficult cases). I had asked him about this particular side-effect and he had replied that the incidence was extremely low. I explained to Mrs McKeeve that all medication has the potential for producing side-effects. I tried to reassure her by stating that the benefits far outweigh the problems. Mrs McKeeve left holding my very first prescription as an independent prescriber.

The next patient I had identified from the doctor's notes was someone who had not had a scan despite suffering a broken wrist while on holiday in England. This 70 year-old patient had 'fallen through the loop' since, anyone of that age who has sustained a fracture would normally be sent for a bone scan to check for osteoporosis. Mrs Lennon was so relieved that I had picked this up since the scan had shown a clear deterioration of her bone structure and she should now be on medication. That seemed like a good result.

I continued with my 'bone' clinic until all the patients had been seen. My next task was to tackle patients who were on an anti-inflammatory medicine but who also had blood pressure problems. What we try and do in this case is to either give the safest anti-inflammatory medicine for pain or persuade the patient to go onto paracetamol regularly and just use the stronger medication for flare-ups.

My first patient was in an argumentative mood. 'My daughter's a pharmacist you know,' she said, 'and she hasn't mentioned any of this.' 'Tell you what,' I said, 'I won't change any of your medication just now, but I'll give you a note of what I plan to do and you can show it to your daughter.' That patient headed off with a promise to come back next week to see me. When she returned, her daughter had explained to her mother that the latest research had recommended one of the older anti-inflammatory medicines was safer in patients with heart disease. So I had won my case and prescribed her new medication.

I looked at patients on certain blood pressure tablets and with any changes I made I obtained the help of the practice nurse to monitor these patients over the next few months. The staff at the practice were critical to the success of the clinics. Whether it was the practice manager searching the computer to identify the patients, or receptionists making the phone calls to get the patients to come for appointments, or the practice nurse taking bloods and performing blood pressure checks – what a team!

The last piece of work I did in that practice was an audit of antibiotic use. This was a check on which antibiotics were being used for patients, for how long and at what dose. The world is now using too many antibiotics. Resistance is emerging with the formation of superbugs with antibiotics being less effective. The first thing I had to do was interview the doctors to find out their views on antibiotic prescribing. A couple of examples of questions were: 'Do you think that too many antibiotics are being prescribed generally?' and 'Are you ever pressurised by patients into prescribing an antibiotic prematurely?'

Obviously, admitting that your own prescribing is not excellent was very difficult but the proof was going to be in the audit. I checked the number of antibiotics prescribed in one particular week in the surgery. I looked at what it was given for, the length of treatment and the dose – the strength of the antibiotic. I then gave all the doctors the latest guidelines from the health board on antibiotics and waited to see what would happen when I looked at their prescribing again.

It was time for the results. The practice manager had arranged for all the partners to assemble in the meeting room. I had put a few slides on my laptop and started with what I thought was quite an amusing comment. 'You've all done very well,' thinking of the television programme 'Are you being served?' The partners were obviously too young or didn't find it funny so no-one laughed and I quickly carried on with the presentation. The results had been good with most prescribing being in-line with guidelines. There were one or two arguments such as 'I refuse to just give three days supply of antibiotics to women with urinary tract infections since they just come back and see me again.' With that one concession, all the GPs agreed it had been a worthwhile exercise and I left them with a congratulatory nod and a written copy of the audit.

The future for independent prescribing in the pharmacy, I think, depends on what medical information about the patient is available, so that the pharmacist can make informed choices. There are now pharmacist prescribing clinics all over the UK.

In 2013 I am prescribing varenicline for patients who are looking for help after a failed attempt at stopping smoking while trying a course of NRT (nicotine replacement therapy).

CHAPTER 8
RESIDENTIAL HOMES

Community pharmacists are involved in supplying medication and giving advice on safe storage to staff at residential and nursing homes.

'I'd like you to do some staff training Mrs Roddick.' said the head of home at Marr Lodge. 'Yes, that's fine but I need to know the levels of training of your staff members and how many there will be on the night.'

Marr Lodge was a privately owned residential home for approximately twenty residents. It was accommodated in a large sandstone villa set in the heart of Newlands just along the road from the pharmacy.

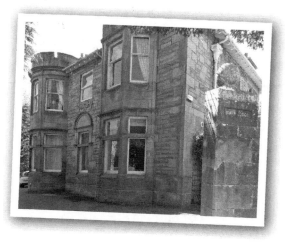

Marr Lodge

After receiving the information I needed, we agreed that I would come along the following Thursday. There were going to be nineteen members of staff. I like to start the training with a bit of a controversial question:' Right, put up your right hand if you take drugs!'

A quarter of the staff members tentatively put up a hand. I quickly put them out of their misery by asking them to keep their hands up if they drank coffee.'Now put your left hand up if you drink tea.' I added. By this time every member of staff had at least one hand up. 'Lastly put your right leg up if you drink alcohol.'

Everyone was now relaxed and laughing so I was able to explain that alcohol and caffeine are in fact drugs. Also, I added, that medicines are drugs that have an effect either to treat or prevent disease. Keeping the staff members engaged was an important part of the training so I kept asking them more questions.'Can you think of any side-effects of medicines that you have seen with your residents?' 'Constipation,' said Jean. 'Drowsiness,' said Sarah and so they went on followed by a discussion about what we could do about side-effects.

After a further question concerning a resident missing or indeed refusing a dose of medication, I decided to change tack and ask everyone to stand up. 'Now this is the ideal position to be in when taking a medicine.' They were all looking a bit aghast at this point so I quickly added, 'Clearly, if your residents have difficulty standing, then encourage them to sit up straight. Let your residents have a sip of water and ask them to place the tablet in the middle of the tongue and then look down while swallowing with more water.' The training carried on for another half an hour with information given on the legality of medicines and the regulations regarding 'borrowing' of medicines. I was also able to glean information on the staff's own training background so that I could target information correctly. I thoroughly enjoyed the night because the relationship with the home, staff and the pharmacy always changed for the better afterwards since we both had a greater understanding of our respective roles.

The pharmacy dealt with three homes, Scott House, Merrylee Lodge and Marr Lodge. We were dealing with approximately one hundred residents so it usually required a dedicated member of staff to make sure everything was done on time. Three weeks before Christmas this particular year, I took my staff out for a training lunch and, because I realised that we were going to be badly behind in preparation, I asked for volunteers at the lunch to work on both the community trays and the residents' medication the next day, Sunday. Linda quickly put up her hand. 'I enjoy working when there aren't any other distractions,' she said. My pharmacy student Tony then put his hat in the ring so it was decided the two of them would be locked inside the pharmacy for four hours beavering away, dispensing while I checked and got everything ready for delivery. What a relief to get up-to-date.

'You'll have to get this medication to us quickly' said Elspeth, head of home at Merrylee Lodge. When my driver retrieved the prescription from the home I could see why. It was for diamorphine injection, a medication used for the terminally ill. In the 1990s, it was unusual for a resident at this stage of an illness still to be in the home, since normally they would be moved to a hospice or hospital as his or her health deteriorated. With the ageing population nowadays, many residents who have been in a home for several years remain there until the inevitable happens.

Pauline beckoned me towards the bedroom and with a hushed voice said, 'Jessie doesn't have long to live.' I entered the room and could hear the forced breathing that I recognised from before. Jessie didn't have any family by her bedside so I waited for a few minutes to pay my respects. I then signalled to Pauline that I must go and, in silence, we headed for the front entrance door.

The next time I saw Pauline was when I was involved in a medicine check of the drug cupboard. She told me then that Jessie had died that night and that two of the girls from Merrylee Lodge had attended the funeral. They were representative of the 'family' Jessie had known for many years.

There was always something happening with one of the homes so there were many nights where I had to work late to get a prescription sorted out to take round to them. I was thinking long and hard about whether I should carry on with my residential homes when the decision was made for me.

'Scott House is going to close' said Joyce. My staff member's mother was one of the residents in Scott House and that meant Joyce would have to find a new home for her. Being a council-run establishment, it was a council decision to close the resource. A group of the residents' families got together and staged a protest outside the home.

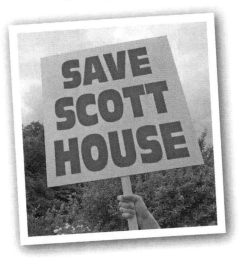

'Stop the closure,' shouted the brave placard-carrying ensemble. The local paper was there taking statements and some of the affected relatives headed into the council offices to hear the official statement read out. The residents have always felt let down by that decision since any arguments against seemed to go unheard.

Marr Lodge was the next casualty. 'I'm afraid we are closing down the unit,' said the owner one afternoon not long after our hearing about Scott House. That meant with all the residents dispersed around the south side of Glasgow, Merrylee Lodge was the only home remaining with the pharmacy. The last telephone call was probably the harshest.

'We're changing our pharmacy to one of the big multiples in a couple of months' said Elspeth, head of home in Merrylee Lodge. 'They're going to give each resident a tray for each medication they are on. It will be much easier for the staff.' It was a very sad time for us because we had been dealing with them for twenty years.

Interestingly, the home telephoned me after six months asking if we would consider having them back again. I did my calculations on what it would cost to give a plastic tray containing individual medication to each resident (that might mean ten trays) and it seemed an enormous expense for the pharmacy to bear so I declined. I often look back on that decision as probably being the wrong one.

CHAPTER 9
CANCER

The lady in front of me at the counter suddenly burst into tears. I had no idea who she was but she was very distressed. 'What's wrong?' I said but I could see she was having problems speaking and in fact was starting to hyperventilate. 'Come into the consulting room,' I said as I led the lady into the back. She was now away from prying eyes. I sat her down and asked her to take deep breaths into a paper bag. When I felt she was sufficiently recovered, I asked Linda to sit with her, while I checked on the dispensary.

'Joyce, when Mr Coslow comes in, can you ask him if he has his yellow book with him?' This book is for patients on Warfarin and has been invaluable in letting all the professionals, the anticoagulent nurse, GP and pharmacist know what dose the patient is on.' 'Yes,' said Joyce, 'but there has been a message from the surgery that they are sending down an American gentleman. He's run out of his medication but the doctor has never heard of the medicine.' 'Fine,' I said, 'let me know when he arrives.' Back to the lady in the room who was by this time quite calm and had become quite embarrassed at the fuss she had made. I signalled for Linda to go back to the dispensary and turned my attention to the lady in front of me. 'Don't worry about that,'

I said, 'no one noticed. Now, tell me what's happened,' I continued. 'I've just been diagnosed with oes... oes...,' She was having difficulty pronouncing it so I gently asked, 'Is it oesophageal cancer?'

The lady looked relieved and started to tell me about how she found out. 'The consultant told us when I went back for my results.' I picked up on the 'us' part and asked who had been with her. 'It was my husband.' 'Where is he now?' I asked. 'Oh he's back at the house. I told him I wanted some fresh air.' I've always felt some people come into the pharmacy to speak to me for a particular reason. Who was this lady and why was she here? I had another stab at what made her come in here and she said she thought I could help her.

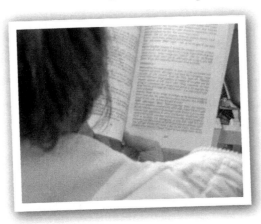

One of the things I do if someone has been newly diagnosed with cancer is give them a copy of a book about beating cancer. One of the topics is nutrition and talks about particular foods and supplementation particularly with vitamin D. I feel that when someone has had the shock news about a cancer diagnosis, then something tangible like being given something positive to read just helps a little at the beginning.

'Excuse me Mrs Roddick', Trish was at the door. 'The American gentleman is here with the empty packet of tablets' 'Right Trish', I said, 'can you stay here with the lady and let me know immediately if things change?' I headed into the dispensary. At this point, I realised I didn't even know her name.

My other member of staff, Yvonne, was signalling to me: 'Mr White is on the phone wondering if his antibiotics could be causing his muscles to be sore.' 'I'll take the call but could you say to the American gentleman I'll just be a minute, thanks.' I got Mr White's computer record up on the screen and realised that I didn't have a note of the antibiotic.

'Hello Mr White', Mrs Roddick here 'when did you get your new antibiotic?' 'It was a couple of days ago Mrs Roddick, my home help came into you with the prescription.' I realised what had happened. Mr White's home help had taken the prescription to another pharmacy and that was why I didn't have the record.

I explained that to Mr White and asked for the name of the antibiotic. Once he told me I could see from his record he should have stopped his cholesterol tablet at night while he was on the course. 'Mr White' I said 'did your doctor not tell you to stop your bedtime medication for a week while you were on these new tablets?' There was silence for a moment then he said, 'Yes he did say, I completely forgot!' 'Right, I want you to phone your doctor and tell him what's happened. I suspect he will tell you again to stop your tablets that you take at night and carry on with your antibiotic but your doctor will give you the right advice.'

After the call I thought now there's a point where if only we had the complete picture in each pharmacy we might be able to avoid problems like that!

I moved out to the front shop. The gentleman in front of me was called Mr Van Allen and as I looked at him I could just imagine him with his stetson hat, since he was from Texas. He was now 75 he told me and was visiting his daughter and grandchildren in Scotland. I looked at the empty packet. It contained two different drugs for hypertension or blood pressure.

'Good,' I said .'What we are going to do is give you two separate tablets because we don't have an equivalent make in the UK. Are you OK with that?' 'Yes ma'am,' he replied, obviously enjoying the attention.

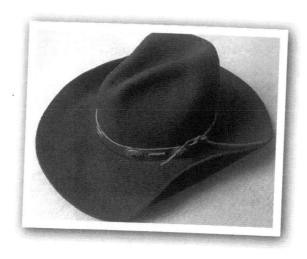

The Stetson

Yvonne got the emergency supply ready and worked out a price. 'I'm afraid I'm going to have to charge you but you can get the next supply from your daughter's doctor if you show him these packets,' I said to the gentleman. He held out his hand and shook mine with a twinkle in his eye. 'It's been a pleasure dealing with your pharmacy.'

'What a pleasant chap,' I thought, 'but help – I've left that lady in the consulting room!' I needn't have worried. She was flicking through the book looking a lot calmer than when she came in. 'I'm sorry, I didn't get your name.' 'It's Rita, Rita Donald.' 'Hello Rita, my name is Elizabeth Roddick.' And so the journey began dealing with someone with cancer.

Rightly or wrongly, I've always felt that the mind plays a huge part in the progression of the disease. By that I mean the prognosis seems to be able to be altered by attitude, personality and sheer determination. It's a very individual preference as to whether someone wants to hear about the holistic approach. There are several techniques that can be used to help the person feel and cope better with their condition. So, after a discussion with Rita, she chose visualisation. Dr Jeremy Geffen has used this technique with his cancer patients so that was the route we took. It involves a series of sessions where the patient decides in his or her own language what would allow the tumour to reduce in their imagination.

Would it be a large garden hose gushing water on the tumour or cleansing the mass in a stream or maybe burning it? It has to be their own language. Rita decided she would take the tumour up into space where it would disintegrate.

Sitting side by side, I asked Rita to take three large breaths. 'I want you to relax and say the words: 'I feel I am inside my body and am attaching myself to the tumour.' I then asked her to describe what she was doing and I could see her face change into a smile when she imagined her trip into outer space. The whole exercise only takes about two minutes so I suggested she did this three times a day.

Two weeks later, her scans showed the mass had decreased in size. Was that just a fluke? Maybe it was, but it allowed Rita to have a few weeks where she enjoyed doing the things she wanted to in reasonably good health. She carried on with her treatments at the hospital but sadly, a few months later, Rita began to deteriorate. Her meals soon changed to liquid substitutes and I showed her the different types, flavours and consistencies of the drinks she could get from her doctor.

It was probably about four months later when I received a call from her GP asking if I could deliver some palliative care medication for a syringe driver that was going to be set up by the district nurse that day. I decided to deliver it myself and I found Rita in good spirits but obviously very ill. The last delivery I did was when the GP felt that oxygen might be a good idea since Rita was having difficulty breathing.

Rita lived up three flights of stairs in a modern flat. There was no lift, so carrying the oxygen cylinders up the stairs was very difficult because of the weight. When the door opened and I saw her son and husband thanking me profusely for bringing the oxygen to them, I knew it had been worth it.

Each person reacts differently to grief. Rita's son was finding it hard to communicate, his eyes brimming over with tears. Her husband, on the other hand, was very matter-of-fact, concentrating on how the dials worked and how to change the cylinder when empty. I said my goodbyes and left them with the difficult task ahead. It's never easy in these situations.

Having dealt with cancer patients over forty years, I've always felt that there tends to be a trigger in peoples' lives before the disease is evident. Stress plays a large part. It could be from losing a loved one, often after caring for that person, ill health, divorce or a car accident. My own brother died of cancer in his early fifties. He had endured a long period of stress relating to his business before he was diagnosed.

But what of the people that survive? Over the years, I have seen so many 'survivors'. There are those who seem to manage to beat the disease. Modern medicine has meant that many now are leading healthy, productive lives for years after diagnosis. I think nutrition is also a factor in beating the disease. If we could encapsulate the thought process that seems to work with survival then perhaps it could be hailed in the same way as a 'blockbuster' cancer drug.

CHAPTER 10
BEING CHAIR OF THE
SCOTTISH ARM OF THE ROYAL
PHARMACEUTICAL SOCIETY

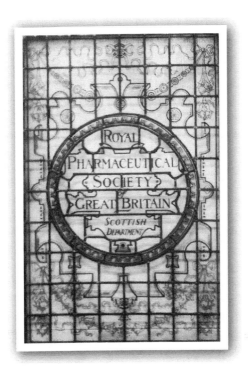

In 1997 I was elected chair of the Scottish Executive of the Royal Pharmaceutical Society. This was the body (now the Scottish Pharmacy Board) that represented the professional side of pharmacy. This was indeed a huge honour and, as I thought, my chance to shape the profession's policy in Scotland.

I did however realise early on that, at that time, the Scottish Executive was inextricably linked to the UK policies through London. My two years as chair were also fraught with difficulties with personnel leaving the office and my oldest brother dying of cancer. However, I had an excellent team of Executive members who carried on with the work of the committee when I was unable to be there. I will always be thankful for their input.

We held our meetings in 36 York Place (now no longer the headquarters) in a magnificent Georgian building purchased by the Royal Pharmaceutical Society in 1884. It was such an impressive building I'm sure it must have been the home of a grand Edinburgh family before it became the office. There was a large brass button on the outside of the ornate entrance and the half-glazed door bore the coat of arms of the society. With the modern intercom and CT cameras, your presence had to be announced before entry was allowed.

The entrance hall had portraits of past secretaries along the wall and the four-storey building had the office staff on the ground floor and the basement was the hall where the AGMs and seminars were held. I remember gathering the movers and shakers of pharmacy together to ask for their help with developing the profession in respect of our public health services.

The library was on the first floor and was available for any member to peruse the literature or research required for study. The boardroom was next and the top floor was the dining room where the caretaker of the day, Ian, provided the committee with a delicious lunch.

The Society also had an interest in numbers 34 and 38 York Place and I believe that my father may have taken his professional qualifying examinations at number 38.

One of the best afternoons I had was welcoming the new young pharmacists to the profession in the presence of the president of the day. I always hoped that some of them would take up the challenge of pharmacy politics and bring their fresh ideas to bear on policy.

The main office of the Royal Pharmaceutical Society was in Lambeth in London and I was invited down for one of the council meetings. I first of all met with the president of the society and, after lunch, attended a full council meeting. These meetings were very formal and had to follow protocol such as standing when the president entered the chamber.

At one point I signalled I wished to speak on a Scottish matter and was given the floor for a few minutes in order to deliver my message.

As chair, one of the things I decided to do was visit as many Scottish pharmacy branches as possible.

These branch pharmacists were the backbone of the profession with many secretaries, chairs and treasurers having spread the word about the work of the profession in their local towns and cities. One of my visits was to the Orkney branch and I must say the trip was one of my most enjoyable. I travelled in a tiny aircraft to Kirkwall airport. I was told that it was going to be windy and yes, when I got off the plane, I had trouble making my way across the short distance to the terminal building.

The branch secretary met me and, after a meal with some of the committee, I gave them my motivational talk about the pharmacy profession and how important grass-roots members were. I was in my element enthusing about the profession and that enthusiasm was put to use when I was granted an audience with the then health minister, Sam Galbraith.

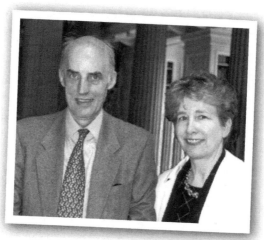

Sam Galbraith at the 50[Th] Anniversary of the NHS

For the meeting, we were summoned to The Scottish Office. (No Scottish parliament building in those days). It was situated at the end of Prince's Street in Edinburgh. This was an austere building with imposing columns at the entrance. Security was very tight and after reporting to the office staff on the ground floor, we had to wait until an appropriate security officer was able to accompany us to the minister's office. This was when we noticed a lot of familiar politicians' faces. I can still remember Alistair Darling's shock of white hair as he passed us in the corridor.

The Secretary of the Scottish Executive and myself had been told we would be given fifteen minutes to state our case so we had prepared thoroughly before going to the meeting. The chief pharmaceutical officer was present in the room at the same time and would ask a question or explain a certain point to the minister if something was not clear. We wanted to suggest that pharmacy could be involved in much more of the public health agenda. The minister listened politely to what we had to say, asked some very searching questions but, as everything was timed exactly, we were ushered back out into the corridor at the end of our fifteen minute slot. It had been difficult to tell how well our meeting had gone except we felt we had used the precious time wisely.

The debriefing was back at York Place and a letter was drafted which, when approved by the board members, was sent to the minister reiterating what was said and giving a possible route forward. I knew I had another chance to state the Executive's case when Mr Galbraith accepted an invitation to come to our dinner later that year. Although I gave a long list of public health services with which pharmacists could become involved, the minister picked up on one in an amusing manner. When I mentioned about pharmacists dealing with head-lice queries independently of GPs in the pharmacy, he scratched his head as an acknowledgement of the issue.

Another interesting evening was when I was invited to Holyrood Palace to meet and have dinner with Princess Anne. There were about twenty-five of us and we had been sent a long list of protocol points before the event. They included how to address Princess Anne, how to shake hands, curtsy or not curtsy and the exact time to arrive at the palace. I remember sitting outside in my car waiting for 7pm to arrive before I was allowed to proceed into the car park.

What a thrill it was going into the Palace where we gathered in an impressive lounge decorated with portraits of the Royal Family and furnished with ornate, antique sofas and chairs. We had all been given a group and area to congregate in and I was delighted when Princess Anne spoke to me about community pharmacy. I made a joke about the fact we have to read what the 'doc' in the Sunday Post recommends so that we are ready with the 'cure' on a Monday morning and she hooted with laughter.

When dinner was ready we were led into a room that had dark wood panelling on the walls and ceiling. We were spread out around the long table and Princess Anne was in the middle, flanked by the chief pharmaceutical officer and an industrial CEO. When coffee arrived, the chief pharmaceutical officer rose and gave a short speech of introduction. It was then Princess Anne's turn and she stood up and delivered what I can only describe as a remarkable speech. Remarkable, since she did not seem to have any notes and remarkable in her knowledge of all aspects of pharmacy, whether it was the branch of community, hospital, academia or industry. Her delivery was compelling and the content extremely relevant, so her advisors also need to be credited with getting that absolutely correct. Our officer alluded to her meticulous attention to detail in his remarks of thanks at the end of her speech. At 9.45 pm precisely, Princess Anne rose from the table, as we all did simultaneously, said good evening and was gone from the room. The protocol was that we had to leave at that point also, so we did, marvelling at the wonderful experience we had all had.

Another exciting invitation I received was to the Royal Garden Party. The envelope bearing the Lord Chamberlain's Officer's stamp arrived that April. The invitation is to the person named on the card and an escort. In times gone by, the partner accompanying the invitee would be an unmarried daughter who might meet her future husband at the garden party. On this occasion, I decided to invite my mother – not perhaps what was expected!

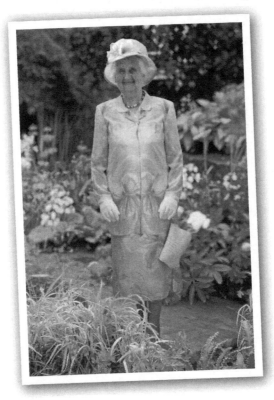

Mrs Betty Ure ready to go to the Garden Party

As I have already mentioned, she was visually impaired and was now registered blind. Because she was unable to stand for any lengthy periods I decided to take her wheelchair with me and use that in the grounds. It wasn't a good day, with rain teeming down as we arrived, so my mother had the obligatory 'rain-mate' over her beautiful powder blue hired hat. (There was such excitement from the staff in the local hat shop, Ella Bulloch's, about the Royal Garden Party, that they had brought several styles down to the pharmacy for my mother to try on).

We managed to get parked fairly close to the gates and queued up with the other excited invitees. As I walked over the lawn pushing my mother, a tall gentleman dressed in the uniform of the Royal Company of Archers – the group of appointed men who guard Prince Charles – stopped me and said, 'Excuse me madam – can I be of some assistance?' 'Yes thank you,' I replied and he took charge of my mother's wheelchair and white stick and placed us at the front of a crowd of people directly down from the Palace entrance.

At exactly 3pm the Palace doors opened and Prince William and Prince Charles moved out of the entrance and stood to attention as the Scottish Regimental band played the national anthem. It was such a moving experience spoiled only by the shrieks of some middle-aged women when they saw Prince William!

As soon as the national anthem had finished, both Prince William and his father moved down the stairs and turned to walk directly towards my mother and myself. Suddenly they were in front of us shaking our hands. I couldn't remember whether I was to curtsy or what. I told my mother that she was shaking hands with Prince Charles and she immediately launched into a story about a mutual friend of Prince Charles and how she, my mother was connected with her. That left me to have a conversation with Prince William, so I started to ask him about his university life and whether he was enjoying being at St Andrew's. He was absolutely charming and a very handsome prince indeed! We then continued the chat across each other, talking with both Princes then, they politely excused themselves and walked onto the next eager couple.

What a memorable experience. I believe my mother was filmed talking to Prince Charles on one of the television channels but we never saw the piece. It had been a privilege to be chair of the Scottish Executive and this experience had further entrenched me in the pharmacy profession.

CHAPTER 11
HEALTH PROMOTION

Is it possible with the right advice, attitude and determination, our patients can take the information they are given and make a difference to their health?

Deirdre was overweight. She wanted help and thought our 'weigh-in' service was just what she needed. Tracey seemed to be the best member of staff to deal with this so we booked Deirdre in for her first session.

It was similar in a sense to the smoking cessation service because the first thing Deirdre had to do with my assistant was work out a goal. In this case she had to lose a stone of weight in four months because that was when she was getting married or rather, remarried. The key to the success of the service is to make a good diet with exercise a 'way of life' rather than 'going on a diet'.

'Have you got your dress?' asked Tracey conversationally. 'Yes' said Deirdre, then she hesitated. 'It's a bit smaller than my size now,' but she added quickly 'I know I'll be the right size by May.' 'No pressure then,' said Tracey as she measured Deirdre's waist. 'What would you say was your biggest problem? What is it that is particularly putting on the extra pounds?' she asked. 'I've got a really sweet tooth so I love cakes, chocolate and juices,' said Deirdre. 'Let's take a note of your meals and snacks in this diary and then it'll be easy to see why your weight is going up.' Deirdre had a BMI (Body Mass Index) of 31 that is termed clinically obese. The BMI is your weight in kilograms divided by your height in metres squared. When the diary was filled in, it showed Deirdre exactly what was happening but the good news was that changing just a few things would make a big difference. 'The more you alkalise your food, the less you'll feel like eating sweet items,' said Tracey. Deirdre looked perplexed so Tracey continued, 'You need to start your meals with a salad and have almonds or celery sticks for snacks. Drink herbal teas and for your main meals reduce the amount of meat you have and fill up with vegetables. Remember to drink lots of water,' she added.

Now let's talk about exercise. 'I don't do any' said Deirdre rather shamefaced. 'Do you work Deirdre?' asked Tracey. 'Yes, I work in an office in the outskirts of town.' 'Do you drive to work?' 'Yes,' was the reply. 'Well I want you to park about a half an hour's walk away from your office. Get some good waterproofs because I'd like you to do one hour's walking every day.'

Deirdre looked horrified. 'Deirdre I want you to keep focussed on your goal, wearing that beautiful size 12 dress.' Deirdre left with her 'pack' containing interesting healthy recipes, her goal and her individual plan. Every week, Deirdre returned for her 'weigh-in' and seemed to be making good progress. It was mainly because of her compelling goal for her weight loss that she achieved it in record time. Tracey was delighted and sent her a congratulatory card just before her wedding. We never heard if Deirdre had made it more of a way of life.

In 2013, every pharmacy in Scotland offers a smoking cessation service as part of the national contract. Greater Glasgow Health Board was instrumental in developing the community pharmacy service and Liz Grant and her public health colleagues led the way.

Things were very different in the 80s and early 90s

A lady came up to me at a social gathering and said, 'You probably don't remember me but I'm sure you saved my life!' This was a very dramatic statement so I was intrigued. She continued: 'A few years ago, you helped me stop smoking. A little while afterwards, I attended an ENT (ear, nose and throat) specialist because I had a lump in my mouth. It turned out it was cancer and he told me if I had continued to smoke I might not have survived.' I did remember that lady. In fact she decided to stop with her friend. That was a great result and I was so thankful to hear that the service had been successful. Many times we pharmacists give advice or perform a service and never hear whether it worked out or not.

It was in the early 90s when I approached the health board for some funding to see if I could try offering a smoking cessation service in the pharmacy. I'd persuaded three of my colleagues in other parts of the city to take part, so, with a little bit of resource, I set up my 'stall' in the corridor at the back of the pharmacy. I had managed to get hold of some charts that showed how many years it would take to get back to normal 'heart health' and how much money someone would save if they stopped for one week, one month or a year.

I placed a notice in the window and all the staff members were primed to let me know if anyone was interested. Yes, my first lady appeared. 'I would like to give it a go' she said. I was treading new ground. Would I remember what to say? What if she asked a difficult question? All of these doubts were going through my mind when I started the consultation. After getting the formalities of name, address and contact number out of the way, I started the consultation. She wanted to be called Jean. 'Well Jean', I said 'when did you start smoking?' I could see she was trying to work it out. 'Maybe it's easier if you tell me at what age you started.' 'Oh that's easy,' she said, 'I remember it was my seventeenth birthday because my friend had bought a pack of ten before my party and asked if I wanted to have a go.' 'Did you enjoy your first cigarette?' I asked. 'Gosh, no, I nearly had to cancel the party because I felt so sick but I persevered and here I am now aged forty-seven wishing I'd never started.' 'I want you to remember that first cigarette feeling – we can use it to help you stop,' I said. 'How many cigarettes do you smoke each day?' Some people don't want to admit the quantity so I quickly said, 'It will mean I give you the right strength of patch.'

'It's twenty to thirty a day,' she admitted. 'Good,' I said. The interview was going well. 'So when do you have your first cigarette?' I showed her the options and waited. 'It's first thing in the morning,' she replied. Now, for the fun bit. The health board had given us a carbon monoxide machine so I explained to Jean we were going to test her lungs.

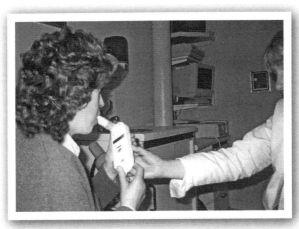

A Patient Blowing into a Carbon Monoxide Monitor

'Take a breath and hold it for fifteen seconds.' She did so and then, as she was going quite red in the face, I asked her to breathe 'nice and steadily' into the machine. At that point, the monitor started beeping and lights were flashing as the gauge started to climb from 0, up and up, until it rested at 22.

Jean looked worried. 'What does that mean?' she asked anxiously. 'It means that your oxygen has 22 parts per million of carbon monoxide,' I said, 'It's not good for your health but the great news is when you come back next week you'll probably be down at one or two.' Jean looked relieved. (The monitor reading is one of the best motivators because the visual memory of the '22' changing to '1' next time really helps the smoker with the attempt to quit).

I then started to ask the 'why' questions. 'What's the main reason for giving up?' as I pointed to the chart with the words health, finance or social. 'It's a bit of both health and finance. I'd like to visit my sister in Canada so the money would come in handy and I know that, with my dad dying at fifty-two with a heart attack, it's probably not a good idea for me to smoke'.

'Yes, keep going back to the reasons for giving up. That will keep you motivated,' I replied. 'Now have you picked a day for quitting?' 'Yes,' said Jean, 'Monday morning will be perfect because I'm not going into work and I go to a keep-fit class in the afternoon.'

'Well between now and Monday I want you to start thinking as a non-smoker. Whenever you reach for a cigarette think about what you are going to do instead. Will you go out for a walk or do extra cleaning? What about after your dinner or when you're on the phone? Get prepared for Monday as you say to yourself, 'I am a non-smoker' and therefore do something else.'

The last thing we had to do was look at all the different nicotine replacement products. 'Would you like to try a patch? This one is the strongest one and you just put it on in the morning and take it off at night. You need to change the position of it in case it gives you a rash.' 'What will I do with my hands?' Jean asked.

'I could also give you the inhalator. The plastic holder looks a bit like a cigarette and when you put the cartridge inside,' (I stopped talking to show her how to do that), 'and then suck it quite hard to get the nicotine out and up to the brain'. By this time Jean was looking a bit puzzled so I suggested she came in on Monday morning and I would put her first patch on and go over the inhalator again.

'Now, lastly, I want to tell you about the three minute rule,' I added. Jean looked intrigued. 'Well,' I continued, 'when you have the urge to have a cigarette, I want you to look at the clock and three minutes later you'll find the urge has gone down. You see why I've asked you to think about alternative things to do?' 'Yes' said Jean.

So that was the end of my first smoking cessation counselling session. Did Jean stop? Yes, for about six months after the initial twelve weeks of the service then a family accident meant: 'I just asked my friend for a cigarette and it all started again.' 'But what did the first puff feel like?' I asked. 'You're right it was awful but I just kept going!' Jean had another two attempts and to date she has never looked back. 'Yes' she says proudly 'I am a non-smoker!'

A man (probably in his forties) was standing at the counter asking Joan about cholesterol testing. She started to tell him about all the other tests that can be done at the same time including fat monitoring when I saw his hands go up. 'Woah, hold up there! I only asked about cholesterol.' I gave him a leaflet explaining the other services and suggested for a little extra payment it would be well worth getting the lot done. Having read the leaflet, particularly about the heart-attack risk assessment he agreed.

Joan booked him in and my student Derek decided to do the consultation. 'We like to do a blood pressure reading early on,' he explained to Iain, 'so that we can do a second one at the end of the session.' The blood pressure reading was normal.

'If you slip your socks and shoes off we'll check your weight and fat composition.' Iain started to laugh, 'And what's the fat composition going to tell me?' Derek explained that he was checking his Body Mass Index (BMI) as well as his visceral fat. 'These readings tell us a lot about how healthy you are and once I've got them all together I'll give them to you in a report. The pharmacist will then go over any readings that seem out of kilter.' Iain relaxed again. 'I hope you don't mind me taking a pinprick of blood?' asked Derek. 'Well I've never been good with needles,' said Iain as he looked in the other direction.

The results were in and I was called into the room. 'Can I ask you about your family history first?' I asked. 'Well my mother and father are in their seventies and they are both on blood pressure tablets. Dad's been told to lose some weight particularly round the middle.' 'Yes,' I stated, 'that's a risk for diabetes but I notice your waist measurement is spot-on.' I went on, 'your blood pressure is normal as well as your glucose levels so no risk of diabetes but both your visceral fat and your cholesterol levels are above average. That means your diet and maybe your alcohol intake need to be looked at.' 'Oh,' he said, 'I wondered when alcohol was going to come into the picture.' I told him about the safe limits of alcohol – 21units per week for a man and he nodded. (I've found over the years asking someone how many units they drink rarely gets a true answer!). He continued to quiz me on the visceral fat reading and I explained that it was 'hidden' fat round the organs.

'Now if you go to your GP they will redo the cholesterol test and if it's high they will probably suggest prescribing you a statin, a cholesterol lowering medicine.' 'I don't want to start medication' said Iain. 'OK I'll give you a print-out of a diet that may help to get your cholesterol down and, if you manage to increase your exercise, then that might be enough. The problem is your own body produces most of your cholesterol.'

Iain dropped by the pharmacy six weeks later and we found his measurements were much nearer the normal levels so I explained it was up to him whether he went the medication route or not but for now he was doing really well.

Mrs Carswell said that diabetes had been running in her family for years and rather than bother the doctor could she have a test at the pharmacy? 'Yes,' I said, 'come in tomorrow morning and we'll check it out.' She arrived just after ten o'clock the next day and we found her levels were a little high. This was a situation where I suggested making an appointment with the nurse at the surgery so that they could double check. The next time I saw her, Mrs Carswell had been given a strict dietary regime to follow for a month then she was to go back and get re-tested. After her month's trial, she arrived back with a prescription for medication to lower her blood glucose. Her GP had decided that with her history this was the best option.

'Oh well,' she said resignedly 'I suppose I'll have to take these for the rest of my life.' 'Mrs Carswell,' I continued, 'you're one of the lucky ones.' 'What?' said Mrs Carswell with a quizzical look. 'If you hadn't been picked up as having diabetes then you might have had more serious complaints to contend with. Diabetes that isn't diagnosed can lead to kidney failure and even blindness so that's why you need to keep taking your tablets.' I then went on to explain that she needed to take the tablets with or after food and we agreed that that should be breakfast and after tea. 'Thanks very much,' said Mrs Carswell, 'I won't forget my tablets from now on.'

A lady was deep in conversation with Joan when my staff member came over and asked if she could have a vitamin D test. 'Yes, that's no problem,' I said, 'what day would suit?' We agreed it would be the next Thursday and her details were fixed in the diary. Before I let her go, I asked her how she heard about the vitamin D testing. 'Oh,' she said, 'one of my friends came along to one of your talks and heard you saying that many people in Scotland are deficient in vitamin D.' 'Yes,' I said, 'it's the lack of sunshine in the summer but also the cloud cover here in Glasgow. The sun's rays just can't get through.'

Next Thursday arrived and the test was performed and sent away. A week later the result showed the lady had a vitamin D reading of 18.2 nmol/L. 'What does that mean?' she said. 'Well, this is the level of 25(OH)D in the blood. The result is given in nanamoles per litre. In your case you are severely deficient and need to supplement urgently.' 'What happens when you have low vitamin D levels?' she asked. 'Well first of all, it is important for absorption of calcium so low levels can mean bone deterioration. There is also a lot of research out there linking diseases with vitamin D deficiency. One example is MS (multiple sclerosis) and others such as cancer and heart disease. What we don't have is robust research showing that if you take vitamin D then it can prevent some of these diseases or in fact lessen their impact. Nevertheless, I suggest you take quite a large dose of vitamin D for about three months then we'll get you retested.'

Three months later, the test was redone and the lady's 25(OH)D level was now at 94nmol/L. As it was now the summer, I suggested she stopped her supplements and tried to get about fifteen minutes of sun hitting her skin in the middle of the day: 'Just until your skin goes pink and don't let your skin burn,' I warned her. It was October when I retested her level-it was only 38nmol/L and as a sufficient level, according to the government, is 50nmol/L, she started supplementing again. Maybe vitamin D testing and supplementing should be much more widespread.

The two young women were having an animated conversation in the front seating area. Yvonne showed me the note they had handed in. The nurse from the surgery up the road had written: 'Malaria prophylaxis Brazil for three months – thanks'. I asked the girls to come round to the consultation room and when we were all seated, I started asking some routine questions. 'So what is this trip about?' Kim answered, 'We've both finished our degrees so we're going to have a trip to Brazil for three months.' I realised early in the conversation that they didn't have much of their trip planned. 'What do your parents think about your going?' I asked. Both girls stated that their mums particularly were quite concerned about the whole thing.

'Right, what I'd like you to do is come back next Thursday when you've planned your trip and I suggest, to keep your parents happy, book as much accommodation as you can'. I then explained, depending where they were going, we would discuss malaria prevention. For our next meeting, I would print out a map. I continued, 'There are two different preparations for Brazil and each has different price structures. The one with fewer side effects is much more expensive. I'll work out a rough price comparison and then when you come back with your exact itinerary, we can discuss the best options.'

The two girls arrived early Thursday morning and this time they had a pretty good idea of where they were going. 'Yes, our mums are much happier about us booking up the different places – it means they'll know where we are.'

'Right, let's have a look at the map.' With the girls' help we plotted their route and I was able to tell them that they needed to start their anti-malarials ten days into their trip. 'So have you decided which type you are going to take with you?' 'Yes,' said Kim, 'our parents are helping us with the cost of the more expensive ones.'

'Good' I said 'I'll work out an exact price but let's talk about the fact that the tablets are not, I'm afraid, 100% effective. You must avoid getting bitten which means using DEET (a repellent) on all exposed areas. At night, you want to cover up as much of your skin as you can with loose clothing and if you are given nets for sleeping under, then you must use them.'

'Let's talk about sun, sand and s_ _.' They looked aghast. 'Remember girls, you are going on a four month journey, anything could happen. Prevention is definitely the safest option'. They softened a bit after that and we then went on to discuss other preventative options such as sunscreen, first aid and water purification tablets. Lastly, I said to the girls in a half joking manner, 'Send me a post-card telling me you're taking your malaria tablets and having a great time.' It was lovely seeing them heading off excited and well-prepared for their adventure.

A middle-aged man approached the counter. I asked if I could help. He seemed very agitated. 'I feel as if I might have high blood pressure,' he said. I felt the gentleman was very anxious and asked him to have a seat and told him I would check his blood pressure in a few minutes. He told me he was 55 years old and when I checked his pressure in the consulting room, I found it was normal for his age and, having asked him a few more questions about his symptoms, I suggested he got in touch with his doctor over the next few days. 'Just to be sure,' I said.

His reaction was one of sheer relief. Somehow the blood pressure check had calmed him down completely and he departed a different character. A week later he came back in brandishing a prescription. I assumed his doctor had maybe repeated the blood pressure check and found it to be higher this time. Instead the prescription was for a cholesterol-lowering medicine. 'The doctor said I was in good health,' he beamed, 'but because my cholesterol was a bit higher, he gave me a medicine for that.' 'I can't thank you enough for your help,' he added. All I did was reassure him, I thought, but that seemed to have made a difference.

I think the strength of the pharmacy service is that members of the public can just drop in, without an appointment and can get some advice there and then.

CHAPTER 12
PUBLIC SPEAKING
IN MY FREE TIME

Pharmacy is about evidence-based medicine. However, I have always believed in the holistic approach to health. If someone is feeling better generally then that can impact favourably on their health. Changing my own diet, increasing exercise and lowering stress levels certainly made a difference to my wellbeing.

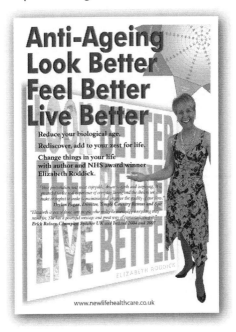

Edinburgh Festival Fringe

Public speaking is a passion of mine although I possibly overdid the hobby when I went along to the Edinburgh Fringe Festival for three weeks in 2007. My subject was anti-ageing and I realised early on that the Fringe is mainly about a pie, a pint and a rude joke. I wasn't offering any of these things, in fact, a large section of the talk was about healthy eating. The young reporter from 'Three Weeks' – the magazine that you have to be in if you want to get an audience – gave me a rave review. The next day the reporter from 'The List' completely slated my show and said she wanted to get out so that she could go for a large cappuccino and a muffin. She also described me as Angela Rippon, as I bounced on my mini trampoline during the healthy exercise section. The average audience at a fringe show I believe is two, so an average of six for me was pretty good. In my naivety, I didn't realise that I could decide on a show lasting only a few days, a week or even two weeks. I was performing every day! Doing a daily show was far too much. Apart from the stress of the show itself, I was trying to run two pharmacy businesses where I not only had staff off sick, but also one of my key pharmacists was unavailable. I would finish the show at 12.40 (lunchtime) and then catch a train back to Glasgow in order to take over in one of my pharmacies.

When one of the technical crew coughed in my face while fitting my microphone to my strap, I knew

I was probably in trouble. Stressed out, exhausted from lack of sleep, it took 48 hours for me to contract a viral infection in my throat and I was starting to lose my voice. By week two, my voice was barely audible and I had trouble swallowing. Of course I had always maintained that the show must go on so I continued to the end of the three weeks.

Three months later, my voice had not returned to normal so, when the ENT consultant said that I had a paralysed vocal chord, I was not surprised. The next thing he said did disturb me. 'There are usually one of three reasons for paralysis, one – cancer, two – a clot or three – a viral infection and I suggest we do a CT scan'. I obviously knew about the scan and had heard many of my patients talking about it but I couldn't believe that this was my going through this procedure.

Thankfully, the scan was negative so, on returning to the consultant, he suggested performing an operation to look behind the vocal chords to see if there could be anything causing the problem. 'Does the paralysis ever resolve spontaneously?' I asked. He replied, 'In some circumstances the chord does return to normal on its own.' Since the proposed operation has a risk attached to it concerning possible damage to teeth, I decided just to wait and see what happened. My waiting paid off and about two weeks later, my voice returned again but it was a very hard lesson. Stop over-stressing my body, give myself plenty of sleep and eat good fresh food, I thought to myself.

The next time I performed that particular talk was at a Southside Glasgow Church Guild. One of the first things I get my audience to do is to stand up and I heard quite a commotion at the back of the large hall. I ran over to find a group of ladies on the floor. 'I held on to Jessie because I felt a bit dizzy,' said the first lady who was called Anne. 'Jessie must have lost her balance and tried to hold onto Betty.' It was a bit like a domino effect, I thought to myself. Obviously, the talk ended abruptly at that point and I offered to take Anne, who seemed to be the most shaken, back to her house with her friend and phoned her son to look in on her that night. I returned to that church a year later to finish my talk, this time with no unfortunate interruptions!

With my passion for public speaking I decided if I was going to be the best, I needed training, so, after a successful spell in a local Toastmasters club, I headed for a public speaking course in London. Part of this particular training regime was learning hypnosis and I was partnered with a young woman called Kate. One of the exercises was to be put in a semi-hypnotic state. First of all, we had to state some of our aspirations.

'I want to feel energetic and healthy and I would like to teach others to feel better as well,' I told my partner. She started to work on the material by setting the scene. She talked me through running along a beach feeling fit, healthy and happy and also got me to imagine being on a cruise ship where I was talking in front of a large audience. When it came to her turn I helped her realise her ambition about meeting her perfect soulmate. We laughed about our proposed experiences but the amazing thing was that, when I returned to my pharmacy, the PR agency which organises speakers for cruise ships had been on the phone and had left a message for me to call them back with my availability that summer. Earlier in the year I had sent a CV and proposal for talks I could perform, but was absolutely staggered that I had had a request to speak.

'Yes I am available this summer' I said trying not to appear too eager. 'We have a slot in August on board the Braemar. It is going on a trip up the Norwegian Fjords,' said Rita from the PR agency.

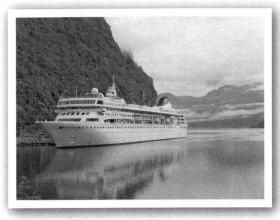

The Braemar Cruise Ship

I was told I had to send a résumé of four talks as soon as possible and she would send two complimentary tickets for the cruise. My husband was amazed as well since the Norwegian Fjord trip was one he had always wanted to take. I came off the phone reeling since I only had three talks prepared. I needed to do a bit of research and decided that, for my fourth talk, I would help the audience find out what was causing the imbalance in their lives and how to get things back into kilter again.

Suddenly, it seemed, August was upon us and we headed down to Southampton with my computer and all the props including a 'rebounder'– a mini trampoline. 'Hey, what are you doing with that?' said the cheery man at the port pointing to it. 'It's to get you fit – would you like a shot?' I replied. 'No thanks' the official said as we were ushered in the crew entrance. We were met by Petra our steward who showed us to our cabins that weren't exactly in the elite section of the ship though very acceptable on the third deck. He was anxious to tell us about one of the perks of being 'crew'. 'You can order any amount of drinks from bottled water to whisky at really low prices'. This was obviously an important message he gave every new speaker. At this point, my husband Douglas was nodding affably, thinking this won't be so bad after all!

The first night, the cruise director gathered all the speakers in a group to talk to us about what was going to happen that night. 'I want each of you to speak for approximately two minutes to 'sell' your talk to the audience.' He went on to explain that there were many competing activities and it was up to each of us to persuade the holidaymakers that our talk was the most appealing entertainment. I was sitting beside one of the speakers who was an expert regarding the Lockerbie bombing atrocity. As Megrahi, the prisoner convicted of causing the incident was about to be released by the Scottish Government, his talk was going to be very popular. Thankfully, it wasn't going to clash with mine.

It was my turn to talk in front of the 300 people crammed into the main theatre. I decided to ask a question: 'Who here tonight would like to learn about the secrets of staying young and improving your memory?' When they shouted out 'Yes!' in unison, I knew I had them hooked.

Over the fortnight's cruise I was told I would do my talks every third day when we were at sea. As soon as the previous talk was finished I had to set up quickly because the allotted time could not be breached since that would then encroach on the act following me. My first talk was scheduled for the following Monday and, as I was setting up, I realised an audience was actually building up. They were coming to hear me and I knew if I didn't blow them away then they wouldn't come to my other three talks. There was one problem – it was quite rough coming out of Southampton. The cruise director had given me a tip – to hang onto a high chair on stage but, as part of my act was bouncing on my mini trampoline, that proved quite difficult. Obviously, the adrenaline was counteracting any thoughts of sea sickness but my unfortunate audience was watching the lecture screen wafting from side to side.

At the question and answer session I thought to myself: 'I'm in trouble,' since a member of the audience had decided to ask questions on her very complicated medication list. 'Listen,' I said, 'why don't I hold a mini medication meeting up in the Crow's bar after each talk and that means people can ask personal questions in a relaxed atmosphere?' And that's what happened, with my little entourage of inquisitive participants.

It was so enjoyable walking along the deck when I had some free time and meeting people who would stop me to ask more questions. 'Can I take vitamin C with my blood pressure tablets or will vitamin B help my memory?' Eventually my husband stopped accompanying me along the top deck and instead slunk along the accommodation level so as to get to the other side quickly.

One evening, we received an invitation from two of the guests who were staying in a state room. 'Cynthia and Donald would like to invite Elizabeth and Douglas for drinks 6.30pm sharp, cabin

1103.' What an experience that was. It was a balmy night and sitting on their balcony as it protruded straight over the water's edge, was the height of luxury. They had invited all their friends from their dinner table and with more questions to answer, we all took part in a lively conversation. 'So do you have to eat sensibly all the time?' said Connie, a friend of Cynthia's. 'No, the key is to enjoy what you are eating and include nutritious food.' I answered. 'Come to my talk on maintaining an ideal weight after the cruise!' Presenting on a cruise ship was an amazing experience and I continue to do my talks to community groups and church guilds.

In my 'Seven Secrets to Staying Young' talk I usually start with slides containing emotive quotations and Louis Armstrong singing 'What a Wonderful World.' I want to get the audience in the right mood before I get them to stand and dance round to 'La Bamba'. This always starts making the audience laugh. Laughter is so important for anti-ageing. Another important factor for energy is the way we breathe – from the diaphragm – that fills the body with oxygen and I teach them how to do that properly.

Eating the right food is critical to staying young and eliminating the foods that age our bodies is also important. 'Is anybody confused about what we should and shouldn't eat?' I ask my audience.

There then follows a lively question-and-answer session involving particular food types.

'What about supplements?' I ask them. 'There are so many on the market that how can you be sure you are taking the right ones?' With our modern foods it is my belief that we do not get all the nutrients we need and supplementing is essential. Trace minerals are lost in the soil and vitamins can be destroyed in storage and cooking.

Exercise is vital to keep the body supple and I explain the benefits of the different types including the one exercise that is guaranteed to make you younger – resistance training. 'I know most of you will not be pumping iron at the gym but you can do the same exercises at home with tins of baked beans or jars of marmalade.' 'Sit in a chair and place a jar or tin in each hand. Now raise them to shoulder height. Do this ten times every exercise session.'

Walking is a great way to ward off osteoporosis and also keeps your mind active. 'Now, if your mind is not in the best shape then very soon you can feel and act like an old person. Some simple techniques such as stimulating your brain by performing tasks that you've never done before can help to avoid that happening to a great extent.' Language can play a significant part in changing mood. 'How do people answer you when you ask them how they are?' My audience usually replies with 'OK', 'fine' or 'surviving'.

'What if you said 'very well' or 'excellent'? Apart from getting surprised looks you will actually feel better,' I tell them.

Short term memory seems to deteriorate as we age, but I say to my audience that people like Dominic O'Brien, eight times world memory champion, improves his memory every year. I teach some of his techniques for remembering peoples' names. 'Have you ever been in a situation where you are standing with a friend and you notice someone coming towards you who you know well? The problem is you can't remember their name and you know you are going to have to introduce them?' Usually this brings a resounding 'yes' from the audience and I go on to explain how to use his techniques on memory.

Maintaining an ideal weight is another talk which features getting back to basics with food. By that I mean eating a percentage of raw food and as much fresh organic food as possible. Avoiding sugar – and that includes hidden sugar in processed food – is probably the best way of avoiding premature ageing. Some races in the world enjoy longevity and do not have our western diseases. Their food is mainly raw, fresh food with only small amounts of meat.

When I give the 'Change Your Life' talks I ask the audience to look at where their life is out of balance. I do this by using the model of the 'Star of Life'. This has all the usual elements of life such as diet, exercise, relationships, finance and career. When all these elements are joined up on a grid they can easily see what is working and what isn't. I realised myself just how out of balance my own life was and, by adjusting things as I stated at the beginning of the chapter, I was able to improve my health in an extraordinary way. Setting out a plan for changing some of the elements, can ultimately mean life is much more in balance. This can be a very rewarding process and many have found it useful as a tool for moving forward.

As well as public speaking, I have a fortnightly slot on Insight Radio as the resident pharmacist. Insight Radio is run by RNIB and is a UK-wide radio station situated in Partick, Glasgow. I try to take topical issues and look behind the headlines as to what is in the research. The headlines are often sensational and putting some perspective on the topic usually brings the research down to earth. I am always looking out for any new research regarding ophthalmic preparations. Early in 2013 I talked about novel ways of delivering medication to the eye.

Simon Pauley runs the Morning Mix programme and likes to start the slot by asking how I am. I always reply, 'Very well thank you,' to which he responds, 'Well you're the pharmacist, you can't be anything else looking after all of us!' It's become a bit of a standing joke!

CHAPTER 13
SUMMARY AND HIGHLIGHTS

In some ways, in 2013, community pharmacy has come back to the way the public saw the chemist shop in my father's day. With the highly successful National Pharmaceutical Association's PR campaign to 'Ask the Pharmacist', modern day pharmacists are as busy answering health questions, providing medicines and screening the public just as they were then.

The profession has, however, moved on in many areas. The public health agenda has expanded greatly. Pharmacy has taken up the gauntlet of smoking cessation services, emergency hormonal contraception, medicine information and minor ailment services to name but a few. Moving from compounding skills to utilising our clinical skills regarding medication has been the biggest change over the last thirty years.

The long opening hours and easy access to a health professional on the high street and where pharmacists have many more over-the-counter medicines available, has meant a bigger role for pharmacy. Nowadays, patients are registering with their local pharmacy so that pharmacists can personally look after their pharmaceutical needs. Electronic scanning of prescriptions means GPs and pharmacists are able to communicate in modern ways. The basis of the pharmacy service is now about patients getting the best out of their medication. The number and complexity of medicines has grown out of all proportion. We help patients use them correctly, for example, taking them at the right time, helping them minimise side effects and giving them all the information they need.

As far as my own life is concerned it has taken a very narrow route in the sense of being steeped in pharmacy but that route has given me such a wide perspective, an insight into peoples' lives, their health but also their trials. As mentioned earlier, I believe in merging the holistic approach to health with modern medicine to help people to feel better.

The whole book contains many of the highlights in my career but I will finish with just three.

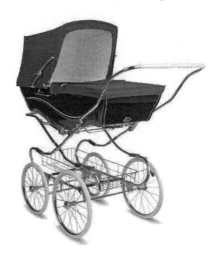

A 1990's Pram

A middle-aged gentleman came into the pharmacy pushing a large pram. He deposited the pram containing his baby son in the middle of the front shop. He had a prescription for an eye preparation for an infection. When I called the gentleman, John, round to collect his child's prescription I explained how it should be used. It was a viscous (thick) drop. 'Just one blob,' I said to him, 'should be placed in the lower lid'. I showed him using my own eye as an example. John looked perplexed. 'Is there any chance you could put in the first bit so I can see how to do it?' he asked.

Here was someone who was experiencing bringing up a young baby late in his own life. He was terrified of doing anything that might harm his precious charge. I looked out at the sea of faces in the front shop who by this time were all gathered round Jamie the baby making strange 'coochoo' noises to keep him amused. 'This is going to be difficult,' I thought to myself. Nevertheless, I donned my sterile rubber gloves and, with the eye drops firmly in my hand, I headed out to do what I thought might be an impossible task.

I looked into the pram and there was the most gorgeous baby looking up at me with wide innocent eyes. I was about to inflict a rather traumatic experience on this child and I had about ten people watching me! There is something about the professional side of life where an automatic reflex takes over. I leant over the baby, pulled down the lower lid and inserted a blob of the preparation. It was a miracle. Not only did Jamie not cry, he actually gave me a huge smile. At this point, the surrounding wellwishers were applauding! What a wonderful memory that moment brings back.

Another time was when an elderly lady came into the pharmacy, kissed me on the cheek and handed me a bunch of flowers. She had come into the pharmacy on several occasions with her son. He explained to me that his mother had been given a medication but she had decided not to take it. 'Could I manage to persuade her?' he asked. The problem was that this lady was profoundly deaf so the conversation was a mixture of sign language, written messages and enunciating clearly in the hope that she could understand me.

I looked at the medication that had been dispensed at another pharmacy and realised I knew nothing about this lady's history. By this time we had sat down in a semi-circle so that I could have as much eye contact with the lady as possible while at the same time gleaning information from her son. I had to first get permission from the lady to discuss her medicine with her son because of patient confidentiality, so that took some time. Finally, she understood and gave me a nod. The tablets were an antidepressant medicine but she was not using them for that so, seemingly after reading the leaflet, she had refused point-blank to take them.

With the help of her son I managed to explain that it was important for her to at least give the tablets a try and I also wanted her to report back to me to tell me how she got on. That seemed to do the trick and that was why two weeks later she arrived with the bouquet. What a lovely surprise!

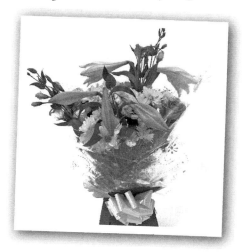

The last example involves my father. His whole life involved making up mixtures, potions and pills so, when I received a request for an old fashioned cough bottle, I thought I would ask him for help.

By this time he was virtually confined to the house because of declining short-term memory. When I mentioned the request, he immediately knew what to do so I decided to bring the ingredients home and let him compound the mixture. It involved heating some of the ingredients in a pan and I wondered how that would have been done in the old days in his chemist shop. What was remarkable was that his demeanour changed, he chatted as he was making the preparation up and for the first time in many months he was smiling.

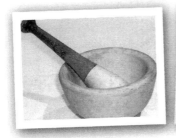 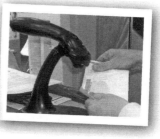

Compounding
Medicines 1938

Electronic Scanning of
Prescriptions 2013

References

(1) Hepler CD. Strand I. Opportunities and responsibilities in pharmaceutical care. AM J Hosp Pharm 1990; 47:533-43

(2) Roddick E. Pharmaceutical Care Plans in a Community Setting. Pharm.J. 1994 Vol 253; 215

(3) Sign Guideline 95 Management of chronic heart failure. Feb 2007

(4) Roddick E. Maclean R. McKean C. Virden C. Sykes D. Communication with general practitioners Pharm.J. 1993; vol 251: 816-819

(5) Wallace M. A Life in the day of... Pharm.J 1994; Vol 253: 215

(6) Yellow Card Scheme MHRA +44(0)8081003352

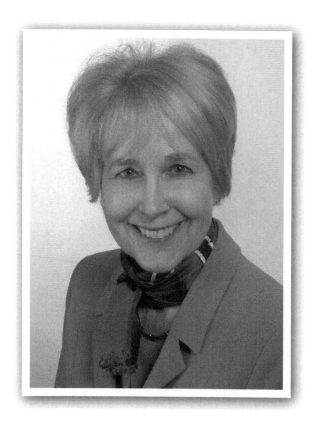

Elizabeth Roddick

About the Author

Elizabeth Roddick graduated from Strathclyde University in 1972 with a BSc (Hons) in Pharmacy and qualified as a pharmacist the following year.

She has owned her own community pharmacy since 1982 .

In 1993 she was awarded the Schering Award for her pioneering work with GPs and in 1999 was given a Fellowship from the Royal Pharmaceutical Society.

The NHS award given to her by the Glasgow Community Council was for outstanding service to NHS patients in Glasgow in 2005.

She has had various roles in the political/professional side of pharmacy and is currently Pharmacy Champion and Community Health Care Partnership committee member for East Renfrewshire, Glasgow.

She works and manages her own pharmacy, New Life Pharmacy in Netherlee, Glasgow. She has a holistic approach to health and she feels her purpose in life is to help people feel better about their health. She is also a qualified life coach and NLP (neuro linguistic programming) practitioner. She lives with her husband Douglas, in south Glasgow.

Other publications from the author can be found at the website www.newlifehealthcare.co.uk